Topological Modeling and Drug Designing

The Author

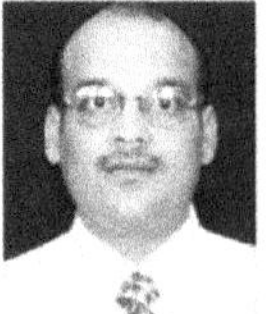

Dr. Dheeraj Mandloi presently working as Assistant Professor (senior scale) in Chemistry at Institute of Engineering and Technology, Devi Ahilya University ("A" Grade by NAAC) since year 2006. He has been teaching Engineering Chemistry, Environmental Studies and Material Science. His area of research includes Environmental Studies and Cheminformatics. He has published several papers at national and international Conferences and Journals. He has attended many workshops, trainings, courses at IIT, NIT, Research labs and Universities. He is life member of Indian Society for Technical Education, Chemical Research Society of India, Indian Association of Chemistry Teachers, Institution of Engineers and Indian Science Congress Association. He is also acting as Reviewer for many national and international Journals.

Topological Modeling and Drug Designing

Dheeraj Mandloi
Assistant Professor
Institute of Engineering and Technology
Devi Ahilya University
Indore, Madhya Pradesh

2016
Scholars World
A Division of
Astral International Pvt. Ltd.
New Delhi – 110 002

© 2016 AUTHOR

Publisher's Note:

Every possible effort has been made to ensure that the information contained in this book is accurate at the time of going to press, and the publisher and author cannot accept responsibility for any errors or omissions, however caused. No responsibility for loss or damage occasioned to any person acting, or refraining from action, as a result of the material in this publication can be accepted by the editor, the publisher or the author. The Publisher is not associated with any product or vendor mentioned in the book. The contents of this work are intended to further general scientific research, understanding and discussion only. Readers should consult with a specialist where appropriate.

Every effort has been made to trace the owners of copyright material used in this book, if any. The author and the publisher will be grateful for any omission brought to their notice for acknowledgement in the future editions of the book.

All Rights reserved under International Copyright Conventions. No part of this publication may be reproduced, stored in a retrieval system, or transmitted in any form or by any means, electronic, mechanical, photocopying, recording or otherwise without the prior written consent of the publisher and the copyright owner.

Cataloging in Publication Data--DK
Courtesy: D.K. Agencies (P) Ltd. <docinfo@dkagencies.com>
Mandloi, Dheeraj, author.
Topological modeling and drug designing / Dheeraj Mandloi.
pages cm
Includes bibliographical references.

ISBN 978-93-5130-966-6 (International Edition)

1. Drugs--Design. 2. Topolgy. I. Title.
RS420.M36 2016 DDC 615.19 23

Published by : **Scholars World®**
A Division of
Astral International Pvt. Ltd.
– ISO 9001:2008 Certified Company –
4760-61/23, Ansari Road, Darya Ganj
New Delhi-110 002
Ph. 011-43549197, 23278134
E-mail: info@astralint.com
Website: www.astralint.com

Laser Typesetting : **Classic Computer Services,** Delhi - 110 035

Printed at : **Sanat Printers**

This book is dedicated in fond memory of

My Mother

Late (Mrs.) Dr. Asha Mandloi

Acknowledgements

It is my great pleasure to place on record the blessings of God which were the real strength throughout the course of the work.

For initiating any assignment, someone must be there whose inspiration leads to smooth working and successful completion. Accordingly, I extend my profound gratitude to Late Prof. P.V. Khadikar, a distinguished scientist and Prof. (Mrs.) Sheela Joshi, School of Chemical Sciences, Devi Ahilya University, Indore for their guidance along with constant encouragements and inspiration during the work. I consider myself fortunate to enjoy the absorbing moments of rigorous academic pursuits in close association with both of them.

My special thanks are due to Prof. A.V. Bajaj, School of Chemical Sciences, Devi Ahilya University, Indore, for constant encouragements. He is responsible for advising me to undertake my work in this fascinating field namely 'Computer-aided Topological Oriented Drug Design'.

I would also like to express my sincere thanks to Prof. S.V. Tokekar, Director, Institute of Engineering and Technology (IET), Devi Ahilya University, Indore and all my colleagues at IET for their kind help and cooperation.

Any flight can reach its destination only with the good wishes and strong moral support from the family members, my mother, father and son Rahul. Special thanks to my wife Mrs. Rakhi for constant motivation and support during my work is very much appreciated.

Dr. Dheeraj Mandloi

Preface

Recently, there has been an increasing need for examining antibacterial and related activities of some important organic compounds for exploring their possible use as drugs in future. This requires screening of a wide range of compounds to investigate the issue in totality along with concern for society. In scientific efforts, there has been desire to look for balance in the efforts and the output without compromising the quality issues. Accordingly, topological studies have recently become more important than ever before.

In keeping with this trend, the proposed book is a modest attempt to quench, to some extent, the intellectual desire of science admirers. This gives an overview of related issues along with details of procedural aspects to arrive at appropriate scientific inferences and conclusions. Suggestions for improvement, if any, are most welcome.

Dr. Dheeraj Mandloi

Contents

Chapter 1
Introduction, Survey and Aim

— A day in the library will save you six weeks in the laboratory —

** Ninad Trinajstic, 2000*

1.1. General

The discipline of medicinal chemistry is devoted to the discovery and development of new agents for treating diseases. Most of this activity is directed to synthesis and analysis of organic compounds to be used as drugs. Organic molecules with increasingly specific pharmacological activities are clearly dominant. Medicinal chemistry is concerned mainly with the organic, biochemical and analytical aspects of the process but the scientists must interact productively with those in other disciplines. Thus, it occupies a strategic position at the interface of chemistry[1].

Synthetic organic chemist has been interested in generating a large number of novel organic compounds which did not exist earlier in the scientific literature as well as in divising new synthetic methodologies[2]. Formation of carbon-carbon bonds is a significant dimension of the synthetic exercise and has attracted conspicuous attention of the organic chemists. The interest has been triggered by exploration of the organic compounds for diverse practical as well as pharmaceutical applications. Friedel-Crafts reaction, Fries reaction, Mannich reaction etc. represent some important reactions in the context of generating new carbon-carbon bonds.

The chemistry and biological activity of organic compounds is very important with reference to our approach to understand their behavior, properties and physiological potential. A plethora of organic compounds are known so that it would be nearly impossible and certainly ill advised for one to attempt to master the subject wearily by acquiring a collection of facts.

Several organic compounds acting as drugs have been synthesized and are excellently modeled using Quantitative Structure Activity Relationship (QSAR) studies[3]. Isolation of active principles, their chemical structure elucidation and synthesis makes an important milestone in the development of medicinal chemistry. With the increasing use of these drugs, many undesirable side effects are appeared[4]. Investigators started researching for drugs with lesser side effects. The new drugs have been synthesized by modification of physiologically active organic compounds. Some new compounds were also synthesized, which have structural similarity with a known compound, which may be natural or synthetic in origin.

1.2. Mannich Reaction and Mannich Bases

Organic chemistry deals with numerous reactions of uncommon and varied applications. Mannich reaction is one such reaction having versatile biosynthetic utility. Mannich reaction provides an important biosynthetic route to natural products like alkaloids and several drugs[5]. This is also evident from the fact that more than 40 per cent researches concerning Mannich bases are published in Biochemical, Bioorganic, Pharmaceutical and Medicinal Chemistry Journals. The Mannich reaction[6] is a classical method for the preparation of β-amino ketones and aldehydes (Mannich bases) and, as such, is one of the most important basic reaction types in organic chemistry. It is the key step in the synthesis of numerous pharmaceutical and natural products. Mannich bases and derivatives such as 1,3-amino alcohols or Michael acceptors, which are easily formed from Mannich bases[6], are particularly versatile synthetic intermediates and find great use in, for example, medicinal chemistry.

The aminoalkylation of C-H acidic compounds was described by several authors as early as the 19th century. However, it was Carl Mannich[6] who was the first to recognize the enormous significance of this reaction type, and it was he who extended the chemistry into a broad based synthetic methodology through systematic research. Since then this reaction that now carries his name has developed into one of the most important C-C bond forming reactions in organic chemistry[7,8].

It is contextual to depict the emergence of the Mannich reaction in the domain of organic chemistry. In fact, the first Mannich reaction (Figure 1.1) took place accidentally in 1912.

Accordingly, Mannich observed that the linkage of two different chemical moieties can occur in one step by means of a methylenic bridge. The main research efforts were of course devoted to the synthesis of pharmaceuticals, and some of them also entered into use as patented products.

Interest in Mannich bases has been quite attractive and wide ranged considering the enormous domain of the applications involving variant nature. While, a large number of Mannich bases continue to be synthesized to explore their biological potential, there is an additional effort to look for variations in the execution of Mannich reaction. A review article has recently appeared which gives elaborate account of modern variant of Mannich reaction[9].

In general, one can use the Mannich reaction as part of tandem reaction sequence for the elegant and often deceptively simple construction of complex target molecule (Figure 1.2)

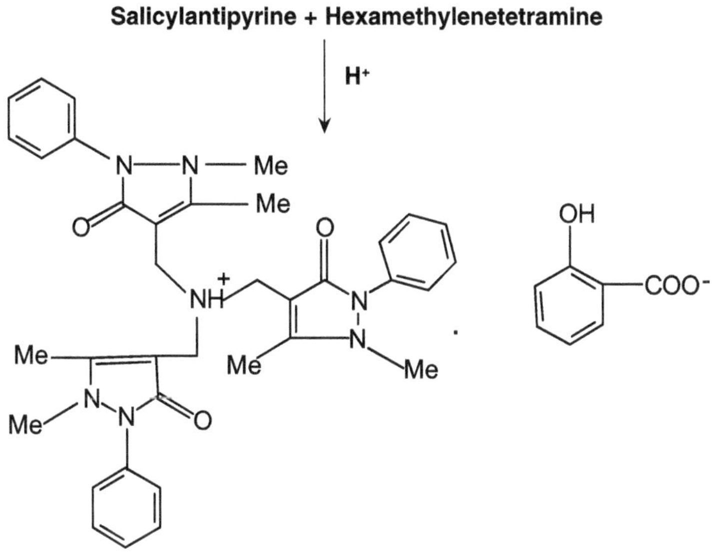

Salicylantipyrine + Hexamethylenetetramine

H^+

Figure 1.1: The First Mannich Reaction.

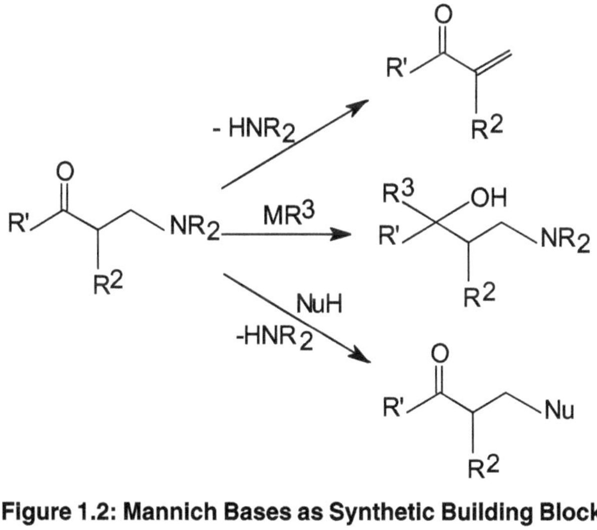

Figure 1.2: Mannich Bases as Synthetic Building Blocks.

Compounds which are enolic, or potentially enolic and also certain alkynes, react with a mixture of an aldehyde (usually formaldehyde) and a primary or secondary amine in the presence of an acid to give after basification, an aminomethyl derivative. For example, by refluxing a mixture of acetone, diethylamine hydrochloride, paraformaldehyde, methanol, and a little concentrated hydrochloric acid, and treating the product with base, 1-diethylamino-3-butanone can be obtained in upto 70 per cent yield:

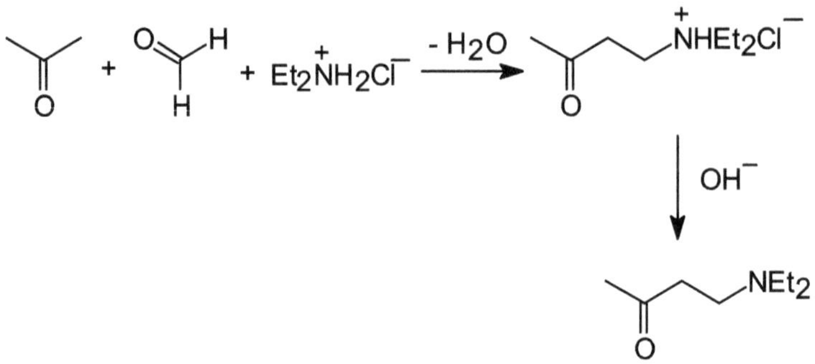

To illustrate the versatility of Mannich reaction[6], it is appropriate to select some of the classes of compounds which participate in the reaction. Each class of compounds has been considered to interact with formaldehyde and dimethyl amine and their corresponding Mannich bases are also shown:

☆ Aldehydes

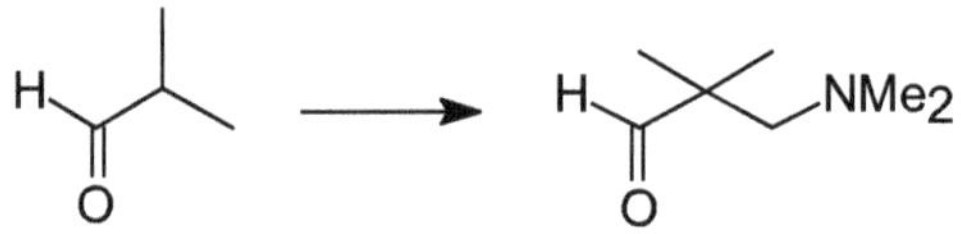

☆ Ketones

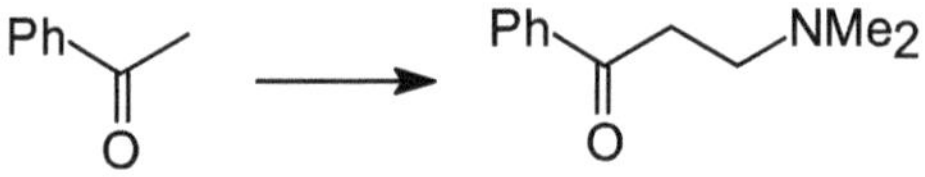

☆ β-Dibasic acids, β-cyano-acids, β-keto-acids, etc.

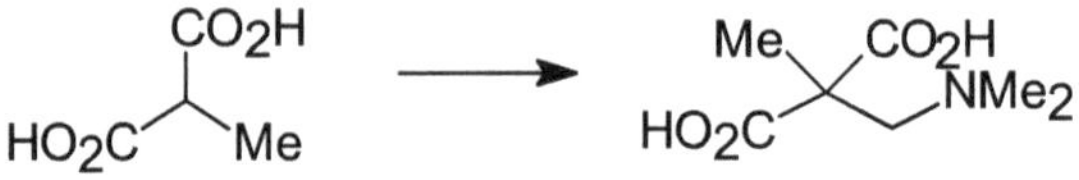

☆ 2-Methylpyridine and related compounds.

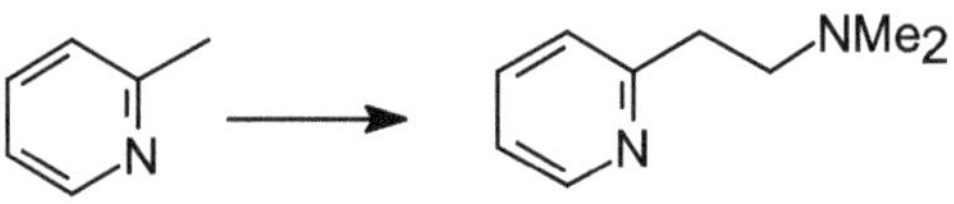

☆ Phenols

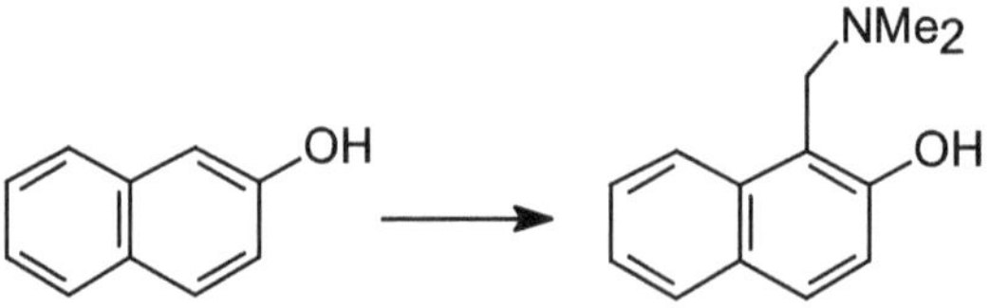

☆ Furan, Pyrrole, indole, and derivatives.

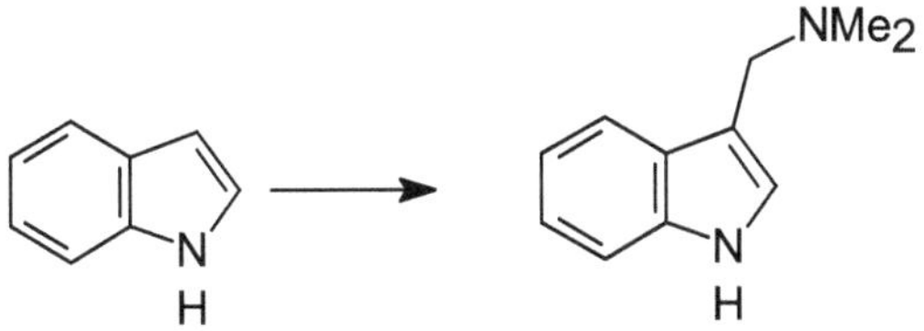

NMe2
N H
N H

While exploring several modern versions of the Mannich reactions it has been noticed that the improved synthetic methodologies rely on ionic chemistry using preformed electrophiles such as imines and/or stable nucleophiles such as enolates, enol ethers and enamines.

The use of a pre-formed immonium salt avoids the need for an acid catalyst and thereby increases the scope of the reaction. The salts can be prepared in general by the reaction:

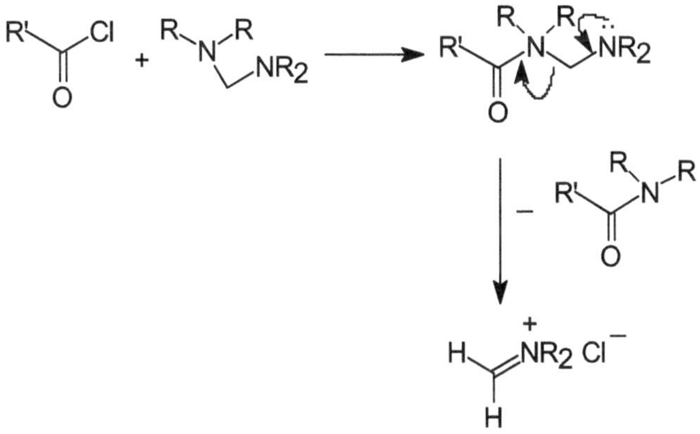

R' Cl O + R N R NR2 → R' O R R N NR2
− R' O R N R
H H +NR2 Cl−

A widely employed reagent is Eschenmosen's salt, prepared by heating the quaternary ammonium salt from trimethyl amine and diiodomethane at about 150°C in tetrahydrothiophen dioxide:

$$Me_3N + CH_2I_2 \longrightarrow Me_3N^+ \text{-} CH_2I\,I^- \xrightarrow{150^\circ C} Me_2N^+{=}CH_2\,I^- + Me\,I$$

Eschenmosen's salt

It is believed that reaction occurs as follows:

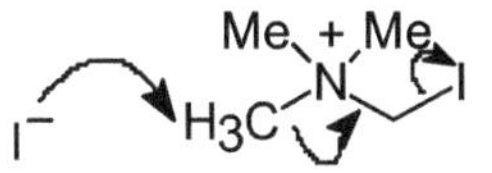

I− H3C Me + Me N I → $ICH_3 + Me_2N^+ = CH_2\,I^-$

1.2.1. Aminomethylation Reaction

1.2.2. Reaction Condition

Formaldehyde is employed in Mannich reactions either as an aqueous solution (formalin) or in the form of paraformaldehyde or trioxane. The amine reactant is used as a free base or hydrochloride. The most commonly adopted solvent for the reaction are alcohols (ethanol mainly, methanol and isopropanol), water or acetic acid. Aprotic solvents or neat conditions are also occassionally used. The reaction is usually carried out by mixing the reactants in equimolar amounts. In some cases, however, amine and aldehyde are allowed to react first and then combine with the substrate. No general rule concerning the choice of reagents and reaction conditions exists; however, a large number of experimental methods are reported in the literature. A more comprehensive survey of synthetic methods, including a description of the experimental conditions is reported[6]; details can also be found in relevant research publications[10–13].

However, under "classical" reaction conditions, with formaldehyde and amine, also, the selection of a solvent can produce important consequences, as found in aminomethylation. Acidic condition are usually adopted in Mannich synthesis in order to favor the reaction, although in some cases, such as in aminomethylation of thiols[14], they serve to enhance the stability of the product formed.

The common procedure for adding reactants consists either in simultaneously mixing all the chemical species involved in the reaction, or in allowing the amine and the aldehyde to react first and then adding the substrate. In some cases, however, the condensation of substrate and formaldehyde is carried out first in order to isolate the corresponding methylol derivative which is subsequently submitted to react with the amino (X-methylation of amino derivatives) compound. This is advantageous with several substrates, such as nitroalkanes[15], ferrocenes[16], sulphonic acid and phosphines[17,18].

1.2.3. Mechanism

The mechanisms related to syntheses involving so many different classes of substrates, the main path of the Mannich reaction are considered only in a general way here[19]. Since the Mannich reaction is a condensation process involving three reactants (substrate, aldehyde and amine), pathways a or b (Figure 1.3) can be followed, if one excludes a rather unlikely trimolecular mechanism:

In the case where formaldehyde reacts initially with the amine (path a), a condensation product having the structure of X-aminomethyl derivative or methyleneimmonium salt is formed, which is then able to attack the substrate RH. Alternatively (path b), a hydroxymethyl derivative is generated, which gives the Mannich base by reaction with the imine. The main points of reaction mechanism are:

- ✰ The relative importance of path 'a' and 'b'.
- ✰ The nature of the aminomethylating species in path a.
- ✰ The manner of attack by the reactive species on the substrate.

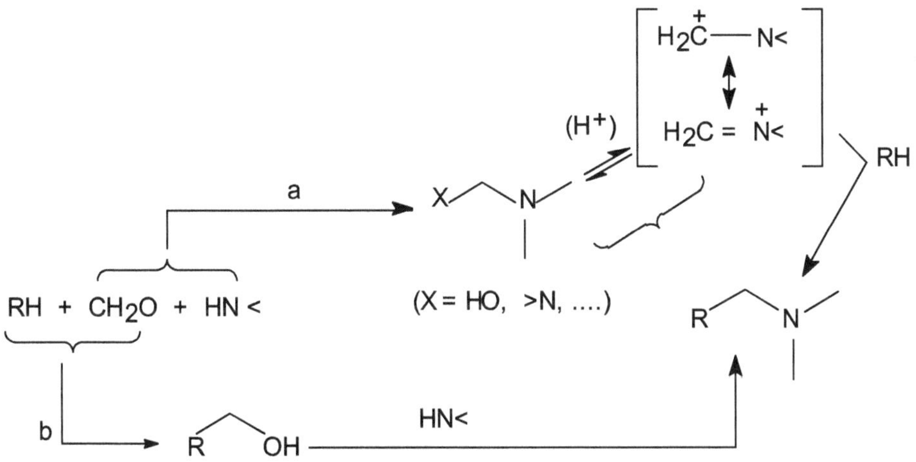

Figure 1.3: Mechanistic Routes of the Mannich Reaction.

The Relative Importance of Path 'a' and 'b'

Path 'a' is generally considered the preferred one, at least when the amine is the most nucleophilic species present in the reaction medium. Accordingly, preformed aminomethylating reagents are quite active, as is well known in performing Mannich synthesis. Indeed, the presence of aminomethylating intermediate has been observed in some cases, mainly by spectroscopic methods. Moreover, the results of several investigations on specific matters favour the predominance of path 'a' over path 'b'.

The Aminomethylating Species in Path 'a'

The actual aminomethylating agent resulting from the equilibrium mixture of (Figure 1.3), constituted mainly by the methyleneimmonium ion, methylene-bis-amine, hydroxymethylamine and in some cases, the ether derivatives of this last species, is an aspect of the Mannich reaction that has aroused much scientific interest[20–22]. Because the methylene-immonium ion is considered to be the most reactive species present in the system, it is usually invoked as the actual reagent[23]. The ion is stabilized by resonance and its presence has been ascertained[24] in the reaction medium under acidic condition:

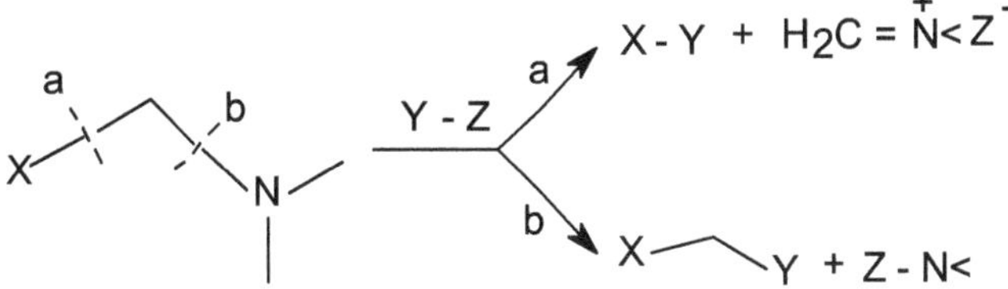

Figure 1.4: Bond Cleavage Required for the Formation of Methyleneimmonium Ion.

The bond undergoing cleavage in the precursor (Figure 1.4) has been particularly investigated in open chain and cyclic N,O-formaldehyde-acetals, since only the cleavage of type 'a' affords the immonium cation leading to the Mannich derivative.

The Attack by the Reactive Species on the Substrate

Herein, the species appears to be strictly related to the nature of the aminomethylating reagent. In an acidic medium, or when a consistent amount of methyleneimmonium ion is present, the electrophilic reaction by the reagent on the substrate takes place[24]. For instance, in C-amino-methylation of the Me group of methyl-nitrooxazoles, kinetically investigated in hydroalcoholic solution, an SE_2 attack by the methyleneimmonium cation upon the substrate has been postulated[25]. When the aminomethylating species is an X-aminomethyl reagent, a mechanism involving the hydrogen bonded complex (ii) is generally proposed for carbonyl[26], phenolic[27] and other substrates[28]. Alternatively, an S_N2 mechanism, involving attack by the carbanion derived from the substrate, has been hypothesized[26–28].

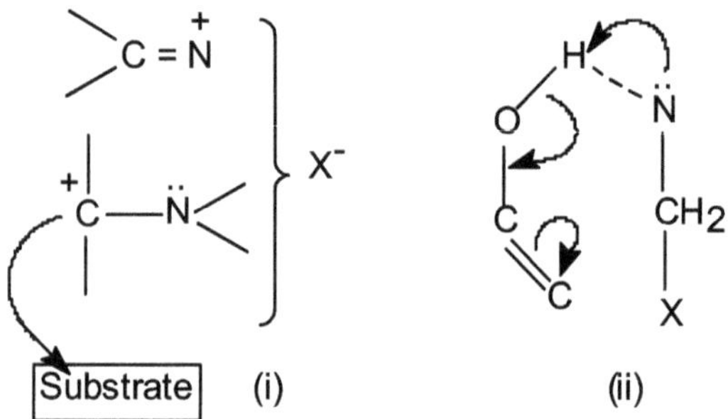

Figure 1.5: Type of Attack on the Substrate by Aminomethylating Agents.

In intermediate (ii) the substrate is considered to be in the enolic form or in analogous tautomeric forms. This assumption usefully clarifies the role played by vicinal groups capable of giving hydrogen bonding with the reagent[26–30]. In particular, the preference for ortho attack observed in the Mannich reaction on phenolic substrates can be explained according to this hypothesis.

The mechanism of this reaction has been the subject of considerable discussion[31–42]. Libermann and Wagner[32] suggested an attractive mechanism. According to them, in general, methylene bis amine is formed as a result of interaction amine with formaldehyde. Subsequent decomposition generates carbonium ion $R_2N^+CH_2$ formed by removal of hydroxyl group from aminomethylol. Since both the routes involve third order kinetics, it is difficult to distinguish between them on the basis of kinetic studies on Mannich reaction in acidic medium. Alexander and Underhill[33] contradicted the mechanism of Libermann and Wagner. According to them, the reaction proceeds with third order kinetics involving no primary salt effect, whereas mechanism of Libermann and Wagner[32] postulates the final and rate controlling step as the reaction between two ions (carbanion and carbonium ion) which should show a primary salt effect. Hence, this mechanism was ruled out[33]. Another possibility has also been suggested of the formation of an aminomethyl ether (III) in an alcoholic medium. A recent study points out that at 30°C practically all the amine exists as methylenebisamine, when secondary amine reacts with formaldehyde[41]. Evidences are available to consider aminomethylether as possible intermediate in Mannich reaction, because the rate of formation of ether is slow as compared to fast formation of methylenebisamine[43].

Verma and Nobles[44] while attempting the reaction with indandione isolated methylenebisamine dihydrochloride. A six membered hydrogen bonded transition state developed during the reaction of nitroalkane with methylenebisamine[35]. The mechanism of Mannich reaction of phenol to account for selective formation of ortho-substituted derivatives has been investigated[37].

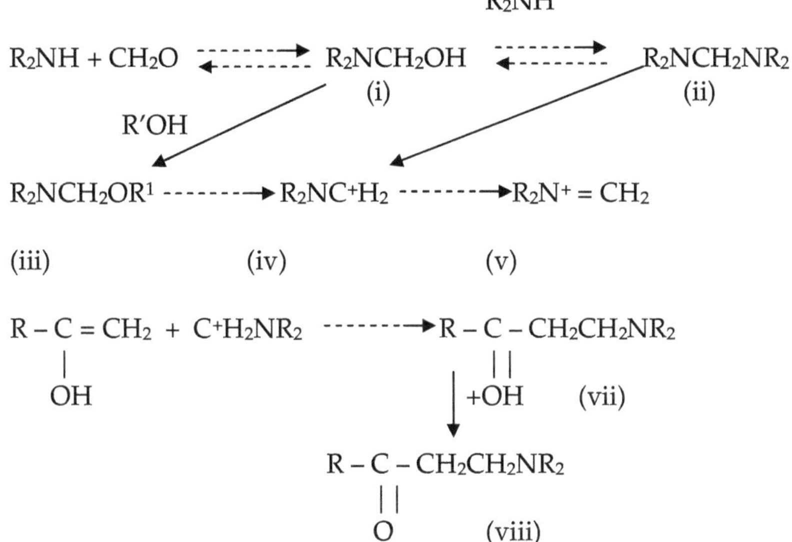

In view of the conflicting evidence in the prior literature, Cummings and Shelton[34] performed kinetic studies of cyclohexanone in Mannich reaction. They postulated that the reaction in basic media involves the condensation of a carbanion, derived from the active hydrogen compound, with an aminomethylol, R_2NCH_2OH, formed from amine and formaldehyde. In acidic media, they suggested that the reaction involves the reaction of a carbonium ion $R_2N^+CH_2$ derived from the aminomethylol or methylenebisamine formed in reaction of the amine and formaldehyde with the active hydrogen compound.

The proposed mechanism differs in that the amine is recognised as being present in equilibrium with the salt formed in acidic media:

Acid Catalysed

$$(R)_2N^+H_2 + A^- \rightleftharpoons (R)_2NH + HA \quad (1)$$

$$(R)_2NH + HCHO \rightleftharpoons (R)_2NCH_2OH \quad (2)$$

$$(R)_2NCH_2OH + HA \rightleftharpoons (R)_2NC^+H_2 + H_2O + A^- \quad (3)$$

$$R^1 - \underset{\underset{O}{\|}}{C} - CH_3 \rightleftharpoons R^1 - \underset{\underset{O-H}{|}}{C} = CH_2 \quad (4)$$

$$R^1 - \underset{\underset{O-H}{|}}{C} = CH_2 + (R)_2NC^+H_2 \dashrightarrow R^1 - \underset{\underset{+OH}{||}}{C} - CH_2CH_2N(R)_2 \quad (5,6)$$

$$\underset{\longleftarrow}{\overset{A^-}{\dashrightarrow}} R^1 - \underset{\underset{O}{||}}{C} - CH_2CH_2N(R)_2 + HA$$

Mannich base

Base Catalysed

$$(R)_2 NH + HCHO \rightleftharpoons (R)_2NCH_2OH \quad (1)$$

$$R^1 - \underset{\underset{O}{||}}{C} - CH_3 + OH^- \rightleftharpoons R^1 - \underset{\underset{O}{||}}{C} - C^-H_2 + H_2O \quad (2)$$

Carbanion

$$R^1 - \underset{\underset{O}{||}}{C} - C^-H_2 + \overset{H\ \ H}{\underset{\underset{R\ \ R}{N}}{C}} - OH \rightleftharpoons R^1 - \underset{\underset{O}{||}}{C} - CH_2 --- \overset{H\ \ H}{\underset{\underset{R\ \ R^1}{N}}{C}} --- :OH$$

$$\dashrightarrow R^1 - \underset{\underset{O}{||}}{C} - CH_2CH_2N(R)_2 + OH^- \quad (3)$$

Mannich base

According to this mechanism, the amine reacts as free amine and not as its salt. Further studies on mechanism of reaction have also been reported[45]. This lead Li and Xiao[46] to make an attempt to investigate mechanism of Mannich reaction involving iminium salt as potential Mannich reagents. They reported theoretical study of the reaction of furan with iminium salt and its comparison with conventional Mannich reaction of furan:

$$H_2N^+ = CH_2Cl + \text{furan} \longrightarrow \text{furan}-CH_2NH_2 + HCl \quad (1)$$

$$H_2N\ CH_2OH + \text{furan} \longrightarrow \text{furan}-CH_2NH_2 + H_2O \quad (2)$$

$$H_2N\ C^+H_2 + \text{furan} \longrightarrow \text{furan}-CH_2N^+H_3 \quad (3)$$

Generally, reaction is carried out with substrate, amine and aldehyde in equimolar quantities. Formaldehyde in Mannich reaction is consumed as aqueous formalin, 1,3,5 trioxymethylene or paraformal-dehyde[47,48]. The amines react as free bases or as hydrochlorides. Solvents usually employed are ethanol, methanol, isopropanol, water and acetic acid. The reaction time varies with the substrate[49,50].

Owing to the unique synthetic potential-perfectly characterised by the title "Mannich Magic" by Heathcock – the intramolecular Mannich reaction has never lost its fascination. Heathcock[8] used the term "Mannich Magic" during a series of lectures given as part of the Merk-Schuchardt Lectureship in the context of the synthesis of the Daphniphyllum alkaloids[9].

1.3. Sulfa Drugs

Since some of the Mannich bases used in the present study are derived from sulfa drugs, it is worthy to make a little comments on Sulfa drugs. This will help understanding the relative potential of sulfa drugs and the Mannich bases derived from them. The sulfa drugs (sulfonamides)[51,52] constitute an important class of drugs, with several types of pharmacological agents possessing antibacterial, anti- carbonic anhydrase, diuretic, hypoglycemic and antithyroid activity among others. A large number of structurally novel sulfonamide derivatives have ultimately been reported to show substantial antitumor activity in vitro and in vivo. Although they have a common chemical motif of aromatic/heterocyclic or amino acid sulfonamide, there are a variety of mechanisms of their antitumor action, such as carbonic anhydrase inhibition, cell cycle perturbation in the G1 phase, disruption of microtubule assembly, functional suppression of the transcriptional activator NF-Y, and angiogenesis (matrix metalloproteinase, MMP) inhibition among others. Some of these compounds selected via elaborate preclinical screenings or obtained through computer-based drug design, are currently being evaluated in clinical trials.

The antibacterial effects of sulfonamides were first observed in 1932, when Gerhard Domagk, a German bacteriologist and pathologist, noted the effects of Prontosil (a red dye) on streptococcal infections in mice. French investigators were first to prove that sulfonamide was the active principle in the dye. American researchers later helped create a rational basis for sulfonamide chemotherapy. Sulfonamides were the first chemical substances that were systematically used to cure and prevent bacterial infections in humans.

They are bacteriostatic drugs; *i.e.*, they inhibit the growth and multiplication of bacteria but do not kill them. They act by interfering with enzyme systems essential to normal metabolic and growth patterns of bacteria. Although more than 5,000 sulfa drugs have been prepared and tested, fewer than 20 continue to have therapeutic value because resistant strains of bacteria have developed.

1.4. Applications of Mannich Bases

Mannich reaction, alternatively known as aminomethylation reaction, has varied applications. Aminomethylation chain introduction in various drugs/compounds has been reported to alter the biological profile and physico-chemical characteristics. Mannich reaction possesses a judicious method for introduction of basic aminoalkyl chain. The various drugs obtained from Mannich reaction have been proved to be more effective and less toxic than their parent antibiotics. Later on, chemists synthesized a variety of compounds possessing potential biological activities[53]. The study of chemistry of Mannich bases has arisen due to two facts:

1. Mannich reaction introduces a functional group by which a molecule can be dissolved in aqueous media.
2. Mannich bases are very reactive and can give many other reactions of pharmacological interest.

Mannich bases have received the attention of various scientists in the technological field. The bases are largely employed as fuel, additives[54,55]. The Mannich bases are useful in metal treatment to enhance corrosion resistance and paint adhesion for metals[56]. The Mannich base derivatives are even used as coagulants[57].

Making use of synthesis and characteristic of a series of novel Mannich bases. Non-conductive polymer fuels have been designed through electro-chemical oxidation of such Mannich bases. Influence of substituents on protectibility of organic coating has been explore in the context of electro-polymerization of Mannich bases[58].

A large number of medicinally active Mannich bases are reported in the literature. They have been confirmed to exhibit CNS stimulant, antiarrhythmic, anti-inflammatory, anti-malarial, anti-hypertensive, antihystaminic antileprosyl, antipsycotic, antipyretic, antitussive, anticholinergic, anticoagulant, insecticidal and antifungal activities. Mannich bass also exhibit variety of other pharmacological properties such as anticoagulant[59], hypoglycemia[60], antiprotozoal[61] etc. Substituted benzamide nucleus exhibits hypnotic and tranquilizer activity of low toxicity[62]. Mannich bases also serve as antihypertensive and antiarrhythmic agent[63,64]. Mannich derivatives from benzoxazoline[65,66], mebendazole nucleus[67], heterocyclic substrates[68], acid hydrazide substrate[69] show anthelminitic property. Several other substrates *viz.*, benzoic acid aminoacetylene ester[70], benzimidazole[71], cyclopentanones[72], naproxen, barbituric acid derivatives[73,74], show antiinflammatory property.

Mannich reaction of benzamide with piperazine, piperidine, morpholine and ethylamine yields bases which are CNS depressant and cardiac stimulant[75,76].

Recently, Mannich bases have been evaluated[77], versus p388 leukemia cells *in vitro* and *in vivo*. Dimmock *et al.*, have evaluated[77] Mannich bases of styryl ketones and related hydrazone for activity against p388 leukemia and significant response towards leukemia cell *in vitro* than *in vivo*.

Mannich bases have also exhibited pesticidal[78,79], germicidal[80], herbicidal[81], insecticidal[82] and fungicidal activities[83]. Some bases exhibit higher analgesic activities and have even proven better than aspirin as in a modified Koster's test[84-87]. Moreover, imidazoline, benzimidazole, nitroxaline, carboxamide derivatives and umbelligerone derivatives[88,89]. New derivatives of Mannich base, Indole[3,2-c] cinnolines have been found to possess antiproliferative, antifungal and antibacterial activities[90].

Researches are going on to evaluate the new synthesized Mannich bases which may have varied applications. Thus looking forward to search some new Mannich bases having biological significance, the under mentioned extension of the field was undertaken.

1.5. Present Study

With the aforementioned information, the present investigation has been undertaken and executed in the following modes:

Mannich bases as synthesized before by the condensation of active hydrogen compounds with formaldehyde and primary/secondary amines[91–102] were used in the present study. The active hydrogen compound may be an acid, phenol, ketone, amide etc.

We have then modeled antibacterial activity of the Mannich bases using topological indices. The used Mannich bases are derivatives of benzamides. The benzamide nucleus also plays a prominating role[103] in exhibiting antimicrobial activity. Various mannich bases of substituted benzamides with sulfonamides shows antibacterial activity with less toxicity than parent sulfonamides[104,105]. The benzamides were condensed with formaldehyde and primary/secondary amines. The primary amines used are Sulpha drugs. The mode of formation can be represented as under:

$$XCONH_2 + HCHO + RNH_2 \longrightarrow XCONHCH_2NHR$$

(Derivatives of benzamide) (primary amine) (Mannich base)

$$XCONH_2 + HCHO + R_2NH \longrightarrow XCONHCH_2NHR$$

(Derivatives of benzamide) (secondary amine) (Mannich base)

The active hydrogen compound was taken in the form of benzamide of:

1. Nicotinoyl-4-aminobenzoic acid

C —NH— C —NH₂
|| ||
N O O

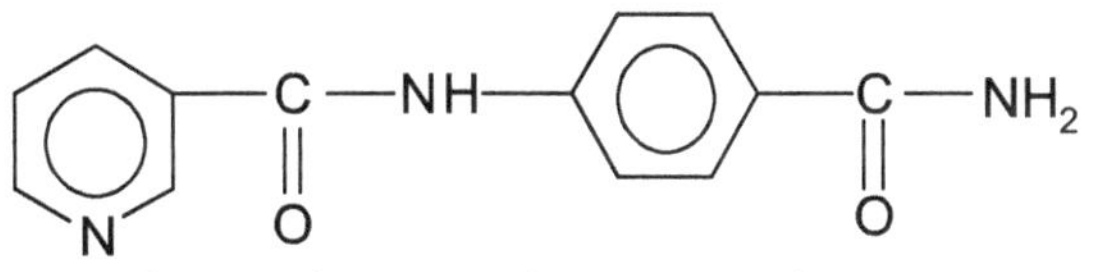

2. 4-Nitrobenzoyl-4-aminobenzoic acid

O_2N— C —NH— C —NH_2
|| ||
O O

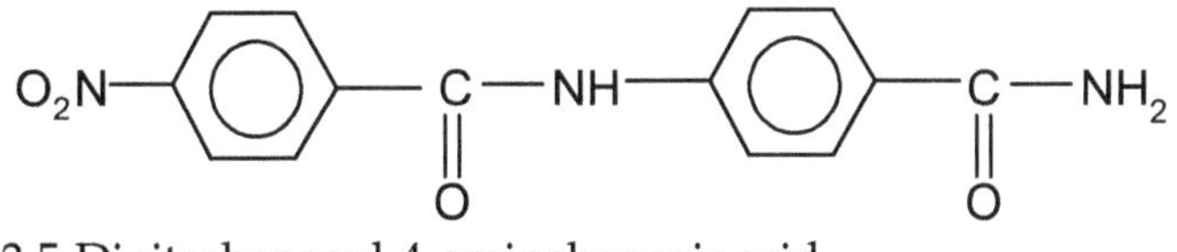

3. 3,5-Dinitrobenzoyl-4-aminobenzoic acid

O_2N
C —NH— C —NH_2
|| ||
O O
O_2N

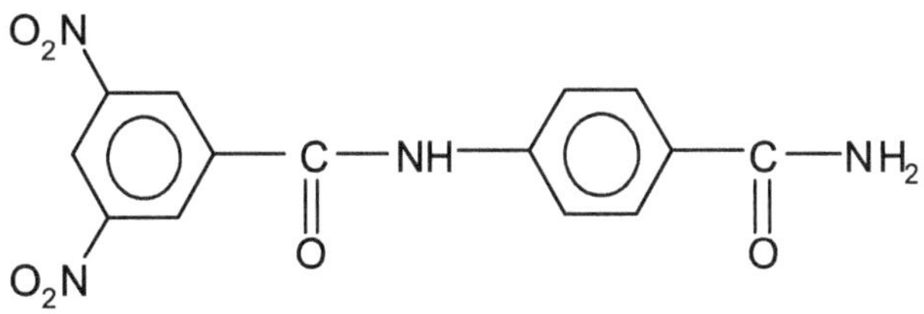

The primary amines were the pure Sulfonamides which are as follows:

1. Sulphadiazine

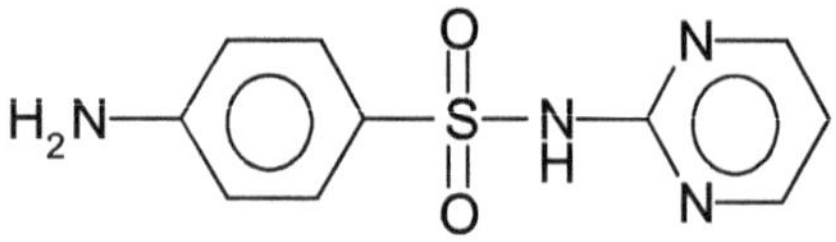

2. Sulphamethoxazole

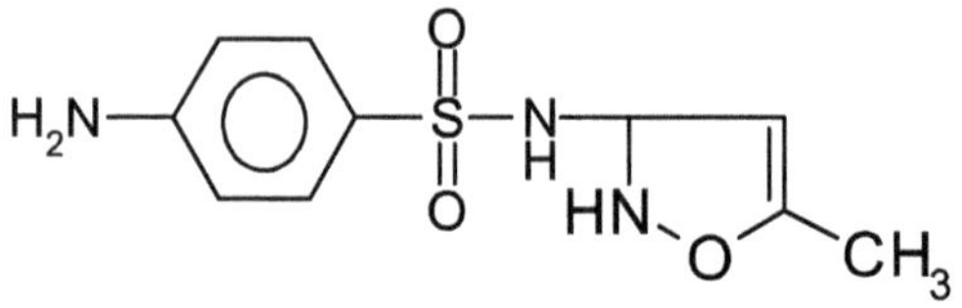

3. Sulphaguanidine

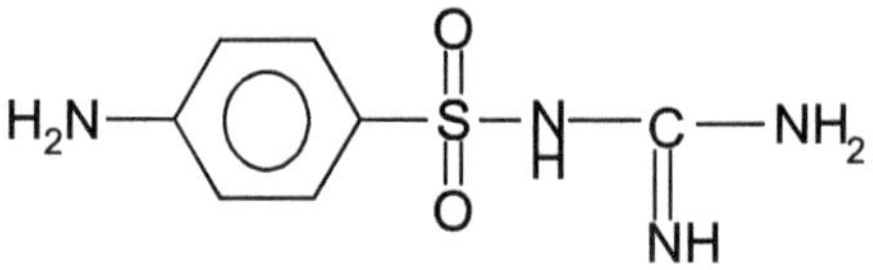

4. Sulphadimidine

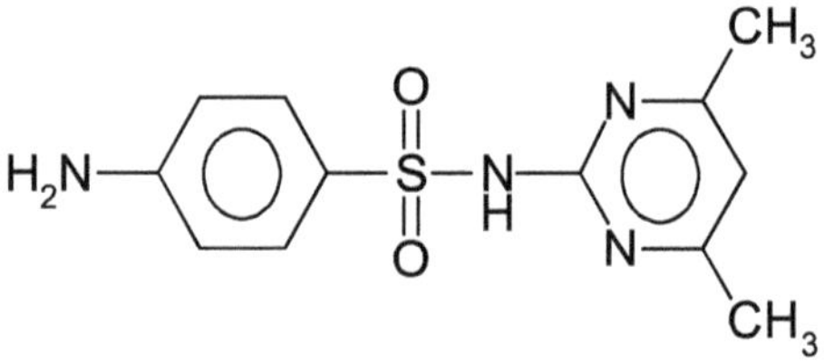

5. Sulphamethiazole

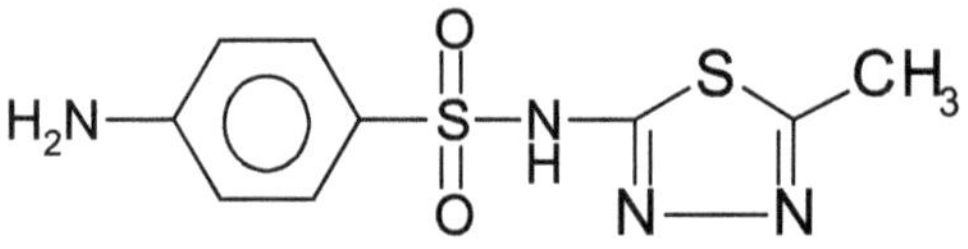

6. Sulphanilamide

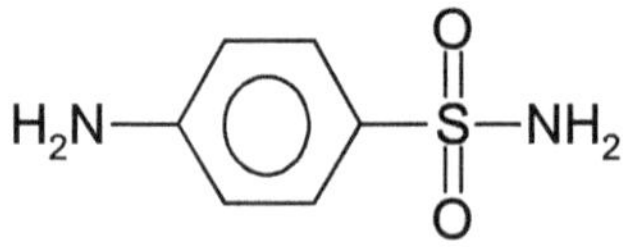

The secondary amines used were:

7. $(CH_3)_2NH$
   Dimethyl amine

8. $(C_2H_5)_2NH$
   Diethyl amine

9. $(C_6H_5)_2NH$
   Diphenyl amine

10. $(C_2H_4OH) 2NH$
   Diethanol amine

11. 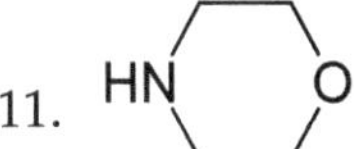
   Morpholine

12. 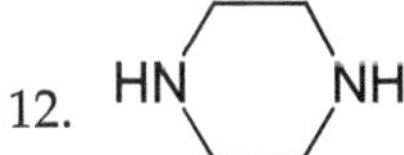
   Piperazine

These Mannich bases were characterized by elemental analysis, uv, ir, nmr spectral studies and screened for their antibacterial activity against some below mentioned pathogenic bacteria by cup plate method mentioned in Indian Pharmacoeipia[106].

Patogenic bacteria used and their patogenicity is given in Table 1.1.

Table 1.1: Pathogens and their Pathogenicity

Sl.No.	*Pathogens*	*Pathogenicity*
1.	*Bacillus subtilis (B. subtilis)*	On occasion acts as opportunistic pathogen, causes eye infection, septicaemia and hemolysis of horse blood cells.
2.	*Staphylococcus aureus (S. aureus)*	Causes cutaneous deep infections like acute osteomylitis, pharyngitis, sinusitis and pneumonae. Causes majority of acute pyogenic lesions in man, causes sepsis in wounds and burns. Contamination in foods leads to diarrhoea and vomitting.
3.	*Escherichia coli (E. coli)*	Causes three main types of clinical syndromes – diarrhoea, urinary tract infections, pyogenic infection including peritonitis, cholecystisis, meningitis, septicaemia and so on.
4.	*Salmonella typhosa (S. typhosa)*	Intracellular parasite usually but not invariably confined to man. Causes enteric fever (typhoid) leading to complications like intestinal perforations, haemorrhage, circulatory collapse, hemolytic anemia, abscess etc. Septicaemia with or without focal superlative lesions.
5.	*Klebsiella pneumonae (K. pneumonae)*	Frequently causes urinary tract infections like abscesses, meningitis and septicaemia. *K. pneumoniae* in rare, but serious disease causing 80 per cent fatality if untreated. It is characterized by massive mucoid, inflammatory exudate of lobular distribution involving one or more lobes of liver.
6.	*Pseudomonas aeruginosa (P. aeruginosa)*	Most common contaminant of inhalation therapy equipment. This equipment has seeded many serious lung infections. It is also a frequent and fatal opportunist in the exposed tissue of burn patients.

QSAR modeling is performed on the anti-bacterial activity of Mannich bases using regression analysis employing the maximum R2method[107] while the predictive power of the proposed models were examined by the Quality factor[108]. The results are discussed in subsequent chapters in that variety of statistics are employed.

References and Notes

1. Joshi, S. and Khosla, N. *Acta Pharma*, **1998**, *48*, 55-61.
2. Hellmann, H., Opitz, G., *α-Amino alkylierung*, Verlag Chemie, Weinheim, **1960**.
3. Burger, A. Medicinal Chemistry, 4th ed., **1994**, John Wiley and Sons, New York.
4. Carson, J.L., Brian, L.S. and Duff, A., *Ann. Of Int. Medicine*, **1993**, *119*, 576.
5. Nobles, L.W., *J. Mississippi Acad. Sci.*, **1962**, *8*, 36.
6. Tramontini, M., Angiolini, L., Mannich Bases, *Chemistry and Uses*, CRC Press, Boca Raton, FL, 1994.
7. Tramontini, M., Angiolini, L., Ghedeni, N., *Polymer*, **1988**, *29*, 771, *46*, 1791.
8. Overmann, L.E., Ricca, D.J., Intramolecular Mannich Reactions: Compressive Organic Synthesis, Vol.2 (Eds., Trost, B.M., Fleming, I., Heathcock, C.H.), Pergamon, Oxford, **1991**, 1007.
9. Arend, M., Westermann, B. and Risch, N., *Angew. Chem. Int. Ed. Engl.*, **1998**, *37*, 1044-1070.
10. Hosomi, A., Iijima, S., and Sakurai, H.A., *Tetrahedron Lett.*, **1982**, *23*, 547.
11. Hester, J.B., *J. Org. Chem.*, **1979**, *44*, 4165.
12. Bohme, H. and Sickmuller, A., *Chem. Ber.*, **1977**, *110*, 208.
13. Jacobsen, E.J., Levin, J., and Overman, L.E., *J. Am. Chem. Soc.*, **1988**, *110*, 4329.
14. Terao, Y., Matsunaga, K., and Sekiya, M., *Chem. Pharm. Bull. Tokyo*, **1977**, *25*, 2964.
15. Grakauskas, V. and Baum, K., *J. Org. Chem.*, **1971**, *36*, 2599.
16. Dixneuf, P. and Dabard, R., *Bull. Soc. Chim. Fr.*, **1972**, *28*, 38.
17. Messinger, P. and Greve, H., *Arch. Pharm.*, **1978**, *311*, 827.
18. Markl, G., Jin, G. Yu., and Schoerner, C., *Tetrahedron Lett.*, **1980**, 1409.
19. Tramontini, M. and Angiolini, L., *Tetrahedron*, **1990**, *46*, 1791.
20. Griengl, H., Bleikolm, A., Grubbauer, W., and Sollradl, H., *Liebigs Ann. Chem.*, **1979**, 392.
21. Lambert, J.B. and Majchrzak, M.W., *J. Am. Chem. Soc.*, **1980**, *102*, 3588.
22. Alva, Astudillo, M.E., Chokotho, N.C.J., Jarvis, T.C., Johnson, C.D., Lewis, C.C., and McDonnell, P.D., *Tetrahedron*, **1985**, *41*, 5919.
23. Lapenko, V.L., Potapova, L.B., Slivkin, A.I., Varil'eva, E.V., *Izv. Vyssh. Uchebn. Zaved. Khim. Khim. Tekhnol.*, **1987**, *30*, 38; Chem. Abstr., **1988**, *108*, 38260.

24. Mironov, G.S. and Farberov, M.I., *Uch. Zap. Yarosl. Tekhnol. Inst.*, **1969**, *11*, 127; Chem. Abstr., **1971**, *74*, 22305.
25. Jagannadham, V., Sethuram, B., and Rao, T.N., *Indian J. Chem. B.*, **1979**, *17B*, 598.
26. (a) Bourguignon, J.J. and Wermuth, C.G., *J. Org. Chem.*, **1981**, *46*, 4889.
    (b) Matsumoto, K., Hasimoto, S., Otani, S., Amita, F., and Osugi, J., *Synth. Commun.*, **1984**, *14*, 585.
27. Mohrle, H. and Troster, K., *Arch. Pharm.*, **1982**, *315*, 397.
28. Paris, J., Couquelet, J., and Tronche, P., *Bull. Soc. Chim. Fr.*, **1973**, 672.
29. Tychopulos, V. and Tyman, J.H.P., *Lynth. Commun.*, **1986**, *16*, 1401.
30. Curulli, A. and Sleiter, G., *J. Org. Chem.*, **1985**, *50*, 4925.
31. Bodendroff, K. and Koralweski, G., *Arch. Pharm*, **1933**, *271*, 101.
32. Liebermann, S.V. and Wagner, E.C., *J. Org. Chem.*, **1949**, *14*, 1001.
33. Alexander, E.R. and Underhill, E.J., *J. Am. Chem. Soc.*, **1949**, *71*, 4014.
34. Cummings, T.F. and Shelton, J.R., *J. Org. Chem.*, **1960**, *25*, 419.
35. Fernandez, J.E. and Fowler, J.S., Ibid, **1964**, *29*, 402.
36. Fernandez, J.E., Fowler, J.S., and Glaros, S.J., Ibid, **1965**, *30*, 2787.
37. Butler, G.B., *J. Am. Chem. Soc.*, **1956**, *78*, 482.
38. Burckhalter, J.H. and Lieb, R.T., *J. Org. Chem.*, **1961**, *26*, 4078.
39. Burke, W.J., Bishop, J.L., Glennie, E.L.M., and Bauer, W.N., Ibid, **1965**, *30*, 3423.
40. Burke, W.J., Nasutarvicus, W.A., and Weatherbee, C., Ibid, **1964**, *29*, 407.
41. (a) Wagner, E.C., Ibid, **1954**, *19*, 1862.
    (b) Fernandez, J.E. and Butler, G.B., *J. Org. Chem.*, **1963**, *28*, 3258.
42. Feldman, J.R. and Wagner, E.C., *J. Org. Chem.*, **1942**, *7*, 31.
43. Cromwell, N.H., *J. Am. Chem. Soc.*, **1946**, *68*, 2634.
44. Verma, R.S. and Nobles, W.L., *J. Pharm. Sci.*, **1966**, *55*, 1141.
45. Fernandez, J.E., Mones, J.D., Schwartz, M.L., and Wulff, R.E., *J. Chem. Soc.* (B), **1969**, 506.
46. Li, Y.M., Xiao, H.M., *International J. Quantum Chem.*, **1995**, *54*, 293-297.
47. McConnel, *J. Diss. Abst. Int.*, **1970**, *30B*, 5433.
48. Walker, J.F. and Chadwick, A.F., *Ind. Eng. Chem.*, **1947**, *39*, 974.
49. Bohme, H. and Hilp, M., *Chem. Ber.*, **1970**, *103*, 104.
50. Fernandez, J.E., Powell, C., and Fowler, J.S., *J. Chem. Engg. Data*, **1963**, *8*, 600.
51. Silverman, R.B., The Organic Chemistry of Drug Design and Drug Action, 2nd ed, **2004**, Academic Press, New York.

52. Supuran, C.T., Scozzafava, A. and Owa, T., *Curr. Med. Chem.*, **2003**, *10*, 925.
53. Thompson, B.B., *J. Pharma. Sci.*, **1968**, *57*, 715.
54. Cherperk, R.E., US, **1995**, *US* 5, 413, 614.
55. Huang, N.Z., Kolp, C.J., and Sgarlata, C.R., *Can. Pat. Appl.*, **1994**, *CA* 2, 102, 331.
56. Lindert, A. and Wolpert, S.M., *PCT Int. Appl.*, 1998, WO 9005, 794.;Inoe, Y., Sato, K., Tashiro, F., *Jpn. Kokai Tokkyo Koho JP*, **1995**, 0762, 048.
57. Makino, K., Yamada, K., and Nibu, K., *Jpn. Kokai Tokkyo Koho*, JP **1991**, *03*, 265, 605.
58. Maruyama, I. And Miyahara, O., *Jpn. Kokai Tokkyo Koho*, JP, **1993**, *0504*, 955.
59. Safaev, A., Kadyrov, A., Saidaliev, Z.G. and Afanas'ev, G.V., Deposited doc., 1974, VINITI 751; *Chem. Abstr.*, **1977**, *86*, 189803.
60. .Khanna, V., Parashar, S.R., Ladwa, P.H., and Bhide, M.B., *Indian J. Chem.*, **1986**, *25(1)*, 102-105.
61. Hussain, M.I. and Srivastava, V.P., *Indian J. Pharm. Sci.*, **1984**, *46(3)*, 103-105.
62. Parthasarthy, P.C., *J. Indian Chem. Soc.*, **1982**, *21*, 969.
63. Botros, S., Youssef, K.M., and Issac, Z., *Egypt. J. Pharm. Sci.*, **1989**, *30(1-4)*, 419-428
64. Khanna, J.M., Tandon, V.K., Kar, K., and Sur, R.N., *Indian J. Chem. Sect. B.*, **1985**, *24(1)*, 71-77.
65. Bercin, E., Seyhan, E., Okan, A., Ilhan, I. Gazi Eczacilik Fak Derg, **1989**, *6(2)*, 163-172.
66. Bercin, E., Seyhan, E., Okan, A., and Umit, U., *Gazi Univ. Eczacilik Fak Derg*, **1990**, *7(1)*, 5-16.
67. Dhaneshwar, S.R., Khadikar, P.V., Katiyar, J.C., Dhawan, B.N., and Chaturvedi, S.C., *Indian J. Pharm. Sci.*, **1990**, *52(6)*, 261-263.
68. Bryant, C., Crow, W.D.L., Paton, D.M., and Bennet, J.E., *PCT Int. Appl.*, **1993**, *WO9*, 324, 446.
69. Jain, R., Chaurasia, O.P., and Rao, J.T., *Proc. Natl. Acad. Sci.*, India Sect. A., **1990**, *60(2)*, 137-140.
70. Dzhuraev, A.D., Makhsumov, A.G., Zakirov, U.B., Nikbaev, A.T., and Karimkulov, K., *Khim. Farm. Zh.*, **1990**, *24(8)*, 30-31.
71. Kumar, B.V., Rao, A.B., and Reddy, V.M., *Indian Drugs*, **1985**, *22(7)*, 373-376.
72. Kasture, A.V., *J. Indian Chem. Soc.*, **1988**, *65*, 297.
73. Chen, H.T., Jing, Y.K., Ji, Z.Z., and Zhang, B.F., *Acta Pharm. Sin.*, **1991**, *26(3)*, 183-192.
74. Koragaonkar, U.V., Deodhar, K.D., Kulkarni, R.A., and Samant, S.D., *J. Indian Chem. Soc.*, **1984**, *61*, 554.

75. Agarwal, S., Pande, A., and Saxena, V.K., *Acta Pharm. Jugosl.*, **1985**, *35*, 31-39.

76. Einhorn, A. *et al.*, *Ann.*, **1905**, *343*, 204.

77. Dimmock, J.R., Jonnalgadda, S.S., Leek, D.M., Warrington, R.C., and Fang, W.D. Neoplasma (Bratisl), **1988**, *35(6)*, 715-724.

78. Ram, V.J., Mishra, L., and Pandey, H.N., *Heterocycl. Chem.*, **1986**, *23*, 1367.

79. Ram, V.J., Dube, V., Pieters, L.A.C., and Viletinck, A.J., *J. Heterocycl. Chem.*, **1989**, *26(3)*, 625-628.

80. Messinger, P. and Judith, G., *Arch. Pharma* (Weinheim), **1978**, *311(1)*, 35-88.

81. Phillips, N.V., *Neth. Appl.*, 1966, 6410300, Match 7, Chem. Abst., **1966**, *65*, 3805.

82. Jain, R., *Inst. Chem.*, **1990**, *62(2)*, 73-74.

83. Khan, M.H. and Giri, S., *Indian J. Chem. Sect.* B., **1993**, *32B(9)*, 984-985.

84. Pilli, G., Erdogan, H., Safak, C., Callis, U., and Sunal, R., *Arch. Pharm.* (Weinheim), **1992**, *325(8)*, 537-540.

85. Unlu, S., Palaska, E., Erdogan, H., Safak, C., Sunal, R., and Gumusel, B., Hacettepe Univ. Eczacilik Fak Derg, **1993**, *13(1)*, 25-30.

86. Vasileva, E., Notova, L., *Dokl. Bulg. Akad. Nauk*, **1991**, *44(2)*, 37-39.

87. Trivedi, P., Ishiguzo, E.K., Gaud, R.S., and Chaturvedi, S.C., *Indian Drugs*, **1989**, *26(10)*, 545-549.

88. Gadre, J.N. and Raote, P.S., *Indian J. Chem. Sect. B.*, **1993**, *32B*, 679-680.

89. Gadre, J.N. and Raote, P.S., *Indian J. Chem. Sect. B.*, **1993**, *32B*, 1285-1287.

90. Barraja, P., Diana, P., Lauria, A., *Bioorg. Med. Chem.*, **1999**, *7(8)*, 1591-1596.

91. Joshi, S.; Khosla, N., *Bioorg. Med. Chem. Lett.*, **2003**, *13*, 3747.

92. Joshi, S.; Khosla, N.; Tiwari, P., *Bioorg. Med. Chem.*, **2004**, *12*, 571.

93. Joshi, S.; Khosla, N.; Khare, D.; Tiwari, P., *Acta Pharm.*, **2002**, *52*, 197.

94. Joshi, S.; Maskar, S.; Khosla, N., Bhandari, V., *J. Indian Chem. Soc.*, **1997**, *74*, 156.

95. Joshi, S.; Khosla, N., *Indian Drugs*, **1995**, *32*, 398.

96. Joshi, S.; Khosla, N., *Indian Drugs*, **1994**, *35*, 548.

97. Khosla, N.; Joshi, S., *Indian J. Pharm. Sci.*, **1993**, 55, 198.

98. Dhaneshwar, S.R.; Khadikar, P.V.; Katiyer, J.C.; Dhawan, B.N.; Chaturvedi, S.C., *Indian J. Pharm. Sci.*, **1991**, *53*, 207.

99. Dhaneshwar, S.R.; Khadikar, P.V.; Chaturvedi, S.C., *Indian Drugs*, **1990**, *28*, 21.

100. Dhaneshwar, S.R.; Khadikar, P.V.; Katiyer, J.C.; Dhawan, B.N.; Chaturvedi, S.C., *Indian Drugs*, **1990**, *28*, 24.

101. Dhaneshwar, S.R.; Khadikar, P.V.; Chaturvedi, S.C., *Indian Drugs*, **1990**, *27*, 431.

102. Dhaneshwar, S.R.; Khadikar, P.V.; Chaturvedi, S.C., *Indian Drugs*, **1990**, *27*, 625.

103. Gorvin, J.H., *J. Chem. Soc.*, **1943**, 735.

104. Singh, B., *J. Ind. Chem. Soc.*, **1979**, 56, 720.

105. Joshi, S. and Khosla, N., *Indian Drugs*, **1994**, 31(11), 548.

106. Pharmacopoeia of India, 3rd ed., **1985**, Govt. of India, Delhi.

107. Chaterjee, S.; Hadi, A.S.; Price, B., *Regression Analysis by Examples*, 3rd ed., Wiley, New York, **2000**.

108. Pogliani, L., *J. Phys. Chem.*, **1996**, *100*, 18065.

Chapter 2
Topological Concepts Used in QSAR

– A day spent in designing the compounds to be made will provide a gain in overall efficiency in terms of minimizing research dollars invested, maximizing information gained

** Ninad Trinajstic, 2004*

2.1. Introduction

In this Chapter II of the present thesis we first discuss drug design, lead compound, QSAR followed by topological concepts used in QSAR (Quantitative Structure-Activity Relationship). By "drug design" we mean the effects to develop new drugs on rational basis. For that it is needed to detect some biological activity in a group of organic compound acting as drugs so as to serve as a lead. Here the lead is a prototype compound that has the desired biological or pharmaceutical activity but it may have many undesirable characters, the chief among them are high toxicity, other biological behaviour, insolubility or metabolic problems. The detection of a "lead" is followed by molecular manipulation to increase or modify the activity. It is worthy to mention that identification of a "lead" depends mainly on the following considerations[1–10]:

1. Molecular structure of the drug,
2. Behaviour of the drug in the biophase,
3. Geometry of the receptor,
4. Drug-receptor interaction,
5. Changes in the structure on binding, and
6. The observed biological response.

Through this identification only a few drugs reach to the level of clinical applicability.

2.2. Quantitative Structure-Activity Relationship (QSAR)

By Quantitative Structure-Activity Relationship (QSAR) we mean a computerised statistical method which help to explain the observed variance in the structure changes caused by the substitution. In this concept it is assumed that the biological activity exhibited by a series of congeneric compounds is a function of various physico-chemical parameters of organic compound acting as drugs. Once the statistical analysis is performed it shows that certain physicochemical properties are favourable to the concerned activity, the latter can be optimised by choosing such substituents, which would enhance such physicochemical properties. The mathematical and statistical analysis of QSAR data finally helps to reduce the number of educated success in molecular modification. During the mathematical and statistical analysis one has to consider the description of the molecular structure, electrons, orbital reactivity and the role of structural and steric components. Then, the ultimate objective of such QSAR studies is to understand the forces governing the activity of a particular compound or a particular class of compounds[1–10]. It means that QSAR is a scientific achievement and an economic necessity to reduce an empiricism in drug design to ensure that every synthesised drugs which are pharmaceutically tested should be as meaningful as possible.

2.3. Parameters Used in QSAR Analysis

We now discuss the parameters needed to carryout QSAR analysis. Generally, the biological activity of a drug is a function of chemical features such as lipophilicity, electronic and steric prospectus, which are due to substituent and the skeleton of a drug molecule[11,12]. Out of these parameters, the lipophilicity is the main parameter[13] governing transport, distribution and metabolism of drugs in biological systems. It is considered as "mechanistic" descriptor of the drug molecule[14]. The other two parameters, *viz.*, electronic and steric parameters influence the metabolism and pharmacodynamic characteristics of drugs. It is important to mention that these three parameters (lipophilic/hydrophobic, electronic, steric) overlap considerably and, therefore, their use in QSAR is problamatic.

Generally, the parameters used in QSAR can be divided into the following two classes:

1. Those parameters which describe mainly the physical properties of a skeleton. The important parameters being water solubility, partition coefficient, chromatographic of values, molecular weight and surface tension, and
2. Those properties which describe the chemical properties of the drug molecule, such as dipole moment, charge density, electron donor-acceptor properties, Hammett's electronic constants, Taft's steric constants etc.

In addition to the above two types of parameters, with the introduction of topological concepts in chemistry and related sciences we have topological parameters also[15–20]. Such parameters are more useful and meaningful as they are numerical representation of the molecular structure. Also, using topological parameters we can obtain 1:1 correlation between structure and activity/property/toxicity.

Thus, QSAR methodology is concerned mainly with the fact that the biological activity/property of organic compounds acting as drugs are a direct consequences of their chemical and physical properties vis-à-vis the parameters discussed above.

For sake of convenience we summarised in Table 2.1 some such parameters used in QSAR.

Table 2.1: Important Parameters Used in QSAR

S.No.	Parameters	Symbol
1.	**Hydrophobic Parameters**	
	Partition coefficients	logP
	π-substituent constants	π
	R_M Chromatographic parameters	$logR_M$
	Solubility	δ
	Elution time in HPLC	$logK^1$
	Parachor	[P]
2.	**Electronic Parameters**	
(a)	Experimental	
	Ionization constant	pKa
	σ-substituent constant	$\sigma, \sigma^2, \sigma^-, \sigma^+, \sigma_I, \sigma^*$
	Spectroscopic chemical shift	ΔFr
	Resonance effect	R
	Field effect	F
	Ionization potential	I
(b)	Theoretical (Quartum) Parameters	
	Atomic charge density	Î
	Atomic net charge	$q, Q\tau, q\sigma, Q\sigma, q\pi, Q\pi$
	Super delocalizability	S_r^N, S_r^E, S_r^R
	Energy of molecular orbitals	E_{LUMO}, E_{HOMO}
	Others	π^1N, N, π^1Nr etc.
3.	**Steric parameters**	
	Taft's steric substituent constant	E_s
	van der Waals randic	r
	Inter atomic distances	B_1L
	Molar refractivity	MR
	Molar volume	MV
4.	**Topological parameters**	
	Topological indices	Such as W, Sz, J, ${}^1\chi^R$, ${}^v\chi^R$ etc.
	Topographical indices	
	Information theoretic indices	

2.4. QSAR Methodologies

Prof. Hansch of Poonam College is respected as the father of QSAR methodology[21]. It was he who in 1964 help chemists to describe SAR-studies in quantitative terms. Following Hansch several QSAR methods are introduced and chief among them are summarized below:

1. **Free Energy Models**
   (a) Hansch method: Linear free-energy relationship.
   (b) Martin and Kubinyi methods: Non-linear free-energy relationship.
   (c) Free-Wilson method: The first mathematical model.
2. **Statistical Method**
   (a) Discriminant analysis.
   (b) Principal component analysis.
   (c) Factor analysis.
   (d) Cluster analysis.
   (e) Combined multivariate analysis.
3. **Pattern Recognition**
4. **Topological Methods**
5. **Quantum Mechanical Methods**
6. **Molecular Modeling**

In an attempt to obtain quantitative information regarding SAR, one of the following approaches are employed:

1. One can use QSAR methods based on linear free-energy relationships (LFER), which relate the activity with contributions from the free-energy related parameters given above. These parameters are due to the substitutes on the molecular skeleton activity as drug. The constants called regression parameters are obtained using appropriate statistical methods. For that correlation of the activity and the free-energy related parameters are subjected to correlation analysis using regression analysis based on the method of least-squares.
2. In this approach mathematical models other than linear free-energy related modes are used to express the dependence of the activity of the nature and location of the substituent.

Alternative to above and perhaps the more effect approach is the computer-aided topological designing, in that topological indices are used as the correlating parameters.

It is worthy to mention that the approaches (1) and (2) are substituent based and are not based on the structure as a whole. However, the alternative topological approach is a structure based approach and if needed it can be factorized not only to the substituent level but also to atomic level.

We now discuss some of the QSAR methods commonly used in QSAR studies.

2.5. Linear Free-Energy Related (LFER) Method

This method uses some of the free-energy related parameters given in Table 2.1 and subject them to mathematical formulation/manipulation. This method is sometimes called extra-thermodynamic method and assumes an additive effect of variable parameters mentioned in Table 2.1 under category-1. This method is based on the following general expression:

$$\Delta BA = f(\Delta L/\Delta H, \Delta E, \Delta Es) \tag{2.1}$$

Here, ΔBA is the variance in the biological activity, ΔL/ΔH, ΔE, ΔEs are lipophilic/hydrophobic, electronic and steric variance respectively. The above expression can also be put into the following different forms:

$$\log BA = b\,\pi + a \tag{2.2}$$

$$= cpKa + a \tag{2.3}$$

$$= dEs + a \tag{2.4}$$

$$= b\,\pi + cpKa + a \tag{2.5}$$

$$= b\,\pi + dEs + a \tag{2.6}$$

$$= b\,\pi + cpKa + dEa + a \tag{2.7}$$

There are three important models, which are based on free-energy related parameters:

1. Hansch Model,
2. Free-Wilson Model, and
3. Mixed Model.

2.5.1. Hansch Model[21-25]

According to this model, which is due to Hansch the drug action depends upon two processes:

(a) The journey from the point of entry in the body to the site of action,

(b) The interaction with the receptor site.

Based on these processes Hansch recommended the following linear and non-linear dependence of activity on different parameters:

$$\text{Linear: } \log BA = a \log P + b\sigma + cEs + d \tag{2.8}$$

$$\text{Non-linear: } \log BA = a \log P + b(\log P)^2 + \ldots (\pm c\sigma \pm dEa + e) \tag{2.9}$$

In principal Hansch model relates the biological activity (BA) within a homologous series of organic compounds acting as drugs to a set of theoretical molecular parameters, which are supposed to describe essential properties of the drug molecule. The coefficients a, b, c, d, e are then determined by multiple regression analysis. However, the major problem in Hansch analysis is the complexicity of the biological effect involving mass equilibria.

Hansch had applied the ρ - σ - π analysis of various problems in order to correlate the biological activity with chemical structure, more precisely parameters related to the substituents. It serves to guide the medicinal chemistry in further synthesis and testing of hetero unknown drugs with still better drug activity.

2.5.2. Free-Wilson Model

The Free-Wilson model[26,27] is based upon an additive mathematical model in that a particular substituted in a specific position is considered to make an additive and constant contribution to the activity. According to this model a particular substituent at a particular position leads to a quantitating similar effect on the biological potency of the entire molecule according to the following relationship:

logBA = Contribution of unsubstituted parent compound + conbination of corresponding substituent

$$= \mu + \Sigma a_{ij} \qquad (2.10)$$

where,

i is the number of the position at which substitution occurs and j is the number of the substituent at that position, while $\mu$is the overall average.

Free-Wilson model[26,27] is preferred when nothing is known about the mode of action or when the physicochemical properties of the substituents are unknown. Best results are obtained in a series with several positions available for substitution and only if each substituent at any location is present in at least two compounds of the series.

Let us now explain the principle used in Free-Wilson modeling. For that we take the example of acetylemic carbamate possessing antitumor activity.

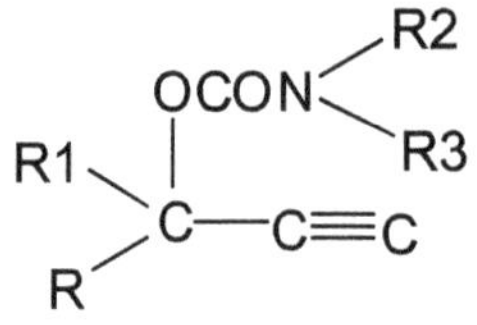

R2
OCON
R3
R1
C—C≡C
R

$$\text{Then, } BA = f(R) + f(R_1) + f(R_2) + f(R_3) + \mu \qquad (2.11)$$

Here, μ is the biological activity of substituted acetylemic carbamate.

Applying symmetry conditions, each components of eq.(2.11) can be solved using the method of least-squares. The active molecule is predicted by calculating the group contribution and by the number of times a particular group occurs in the analysis.

The difference between Hansch and Free-Wilson approach is obviously the former uses substitution constants related to the biological activity while the latter uses physical properties.

2.5.3. Mixed Model: Kubinyi Model

This model proposed by Kubinyi[28] is a combination of Hansch and Free-Wilson model and is given by the following relationship:

Hansch Model: $\log I/C = K_1\pi + K_2\sigma + K_3Es + K$ (2.12)

Free-Wilson Model: $\log I/C = \mu + \Sigma\, a_{ij}$

Kubinyi Model = Hansch Model + Free-Wilson Model

$= \Sigma K_j\,\phi_j + K + \Sigma\, a_{ij}$ (2.13)

where,

K_j represents the coefficient of different physicochemical parameters.

In the above eq.(2.13), Σa_{ij}- is the Free-Wilson part for the substituents and $\phi_j = \pi$, σ and Es contribution of the parent skeleton.

This model is developed with a particular interest to find out possible interaction between Free-Wilson parameters and physicochemical properties of the substituents. The modeling can be applied to a congeneric series having a common skeleton. Therefore, various derivatives must be prepared by using different substituents at the same distinct positions of the parent skeleton. The substituents contribute to the activity additatively at the same position. While choosing derivative for the synthesis, care need to be taken that every substituent appears at least twice at the same position.

The advantages of Free-Wilson approach are summarized below:

(1) It is simple, fast and cheap method wherein no substitution constants like π, σ, Es are needed,

(2) The greater the complexity of the structure, the larger is the number of possible substituents at desired positions. Hence, the efficiency of this approach is high,

(3) At each position, the contribution of each substituent can clearly be identified. The substituents which can or cannot fulfil the principle of additivity, can be recognized.

(4) It is effective especially when substituent constants are not available.

Inspite of the above advantages the Free-Wilson modeling suffers from the following disadvantages:

(1) A prediction of activity increments outside the substituents used in the data set by extrapolation is rather impossible, and

(2) The assumed independence of substituents on the total activity is often not seen in practice.

In addition to these methods of modeling the activity we have some other models, such as mentioned below:

(1) Fujita-Bar Model,

(2) Cluster Significance Analysis,

(3) Discriminate Analysis,
(4) Minimal Topological Difference (MTD) method,
(5) Molecular Orbital Analysis,
(6) Principal Component Analysis (PCA),
(7) Molecular Modeling, and
(8) Topliss Decision Tree Method.

Since our Ph.D. work relates to topological approach, now we discuss "Minimal Toological Difference (MTD) Method".

2.6. MinMinimal Topological Difference (MTD) Method

The "Minimal Topological Difference (MTD) Method" is introduced by Simon and coworkers, 1973 [29]. It relates to the degree of steric misfit of a drug molecule with respect to the receptor site. Minimal steric differences are obtained by comparing them topologically, *i.e.*, shape of newly synthesized drug with the minimal essential parts of the standard clinically used drugs.

The comparison of the molecular shape of the molecules of the drug series under investigation is done by an atom by atom superimposition of the molecular structure yielding a network called hyper molecule. The latter represents partially, the stereo-chemistry of drug molecules bound to the receptor site.

The basic assumption in this method are as follows:

(1) Hydrogen atoms are neglected,
(2) Small differences in bond length (± 0.28 A°) and bond angle (± 20°) are neglected, and
(3) Molecules may exhibit several low energy conformations, out of which such conformation having maximal superimposition with the standard pharmacophore is chosen.

2.7. Still Better Topological Methods

Still better, more effective, and useful methods are those based on topological indices. These topological indices are numerical representation of molecular graph, vis-à-vis molecular structure. In obtaining such indices first the molecular structure is transformed into its molecular graph by deleting all the carbon-hydrogen as well as heteroatom-hydrogen bonds from the molecular structure. In the molecular graph so obtained the atoms are considered as vertices and are denoted by a dot '.' or small circle 'o', while the bonds on the other hand are called edges and are represented by a small line ' – '. Initially, no distinction is made among single, double, triple and aromatic bonds.

By imposing different conditions on vertices (atoms), edges (bonds) and both, a number is obtained which represents molecular structure and is called the topological index, more precisely it is called as graph-theoretical descriptor. A plathora of such topological indices are reported in the literature, out of which only a few are successfully used in QSAR.

Normally topologial indices are obtained from the topological matrices. Out of these matrices the distance matrix (D) and adjacency matrix (A) are more important. However, the important topological matrices are as below and several topological indices are derived from them:

(1) Adjacency Matrix (A),
(2) Extended Adjacency Matrix (E_A),
(3) Distance Matrix (D),
(4) Reciprocal Distance Matrix (D^{-1}),
(5) Decotor Matrix (Δ),
(6) Bond Matrix (b-matrix),
(7) Bond-Electron Matrix (be-Matrix),
(8) Combinational Matrix,
(9) Chemistry Intuitive Adjacency Matrix,
(10) Laplacian or Kirchhoff Matrix,
(11) Layer Matrix,
(12) Shell Matrix,
(13) Wiener Matrix,
(14) Szeged Matrix,
(15) Cluj Matrix, and
(16) 3D-Distance Matrix.

Out of these topological matrices the first 9 are widely used. It is, therefore, necessary to get familiar with these matrices and also to know which and what types of topological indices can be derived from them. This is made clear in the following section. The details of all the 16 matrices and other related matrices are available in the review book by Diudea-Khadikar[30].

2.7.1. Adjacency Matrix (A)

Discovered/introduced in 1874 by Sylvester

Hiickel Matrix is the same as adjacency matrix:

$$[A]_{ij} = \begin{cases} 1 \text{ if } i \neq j \text{ and } i, j \in E(G) \\ 0 \text{ if } i = j \text{ and } i, j \in E(G) \end{cases}$$

Adjacency Matrix of a Weighted Graph

Adjacency matrix can be weighted using the following parameters:

(1) Atom contribution: $D_{ij} = 1 - \dfrac{Zc}{Zi}$

(2) Bond weight (Wr): Single bond = 1, Double bond = 2,
Triple bond = 3, Aromatic Bond = 1.5

(3) Bond parameter: $Kr = \frac{1}{Wr} \cdot \frac{(Zc)^2}{Z_i \cdot Z_j}$

Kr =	
	$C-C = 1.000$
	$C=C = 0.500$
	$C \equiv C = 0.333$
	$(C\text{-}C)_{Aro} = 0.670$

D_{ii} =		
	C = 0.000	Cl = 0.647
	N = 0.143	P = 0.690
	O = 0.250	
	S = 0.625	
	F = 0.33 3	

Atomic Number		
C = 6	S = 16	P = 15
N = 7	F = 9	
O = 8	Cl = 17	

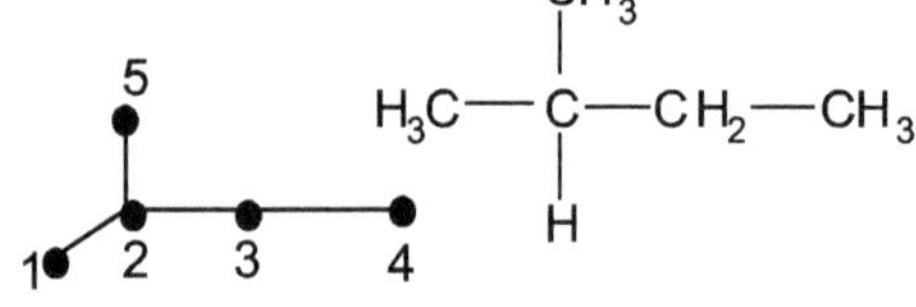

Example: 2-Methyl Butane

	1	2	3	4	5		Entries into degree Vector
1	0	1	0	0	0	1	Gives: Vertex Degree
2	1	0	1	1	0	3	: Topological valency
3	0	1	0	0	1	2	: # Vertices (atoms)
4	0	0	1	0	0	1	following on i.
5	0	1	0	0	0	1	
1	3	2	1	1	8		

Degree vector $V = \{ V_I \} \equiv \{ 1\,3\,2\,1\,1 \}$

Topological Indices Derived from Adjacency Matrix (A)

(Introduced by Gutman, 1972)

(1) Degree Sums: ΣV

(2) Zagreb Indices: M_1, M_2

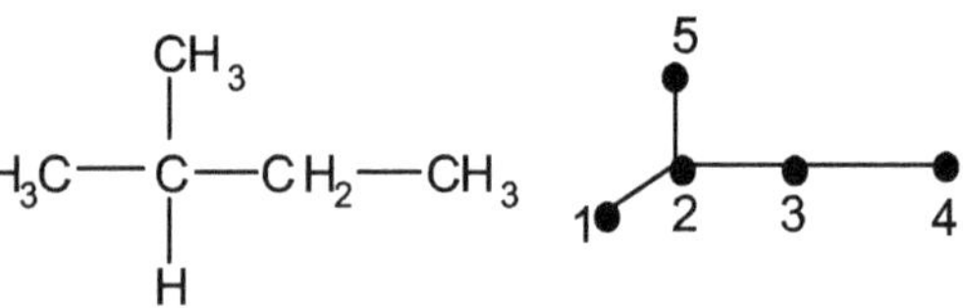

(3) Modified Zagreb: M_2 (Trinajastic 2003)

$v = |\ 1\,3\,2\,1\,1\ |$

(4) Randic Connectivity Indices: $^n\chi$

$M_1 = \Sigma v_i^2 : 1^2 + 3^2 + 2^2 + 1^2 + 1^2 = 16$

$M_2 = \sum_e v_i \cdot v_j : 1.3 + 3.2 + 2.1 + 3.1 = 14$

$$\text{Modified } M_2 = \sum_e (v_i v_j)^{-1} = \frac{1}{3} + \frac{1}{6} + \frac{1}{2} + \frac{1}{3} =$$

Uses of Zagreb Indices

(1) Molecular complexicity

(2) Molecular chirality

(3) Z-E isomerism

(4) Heterosystems

(5) QSPR/QSAR/QSTR

Randic Connectivity Indices: $^n\chi$

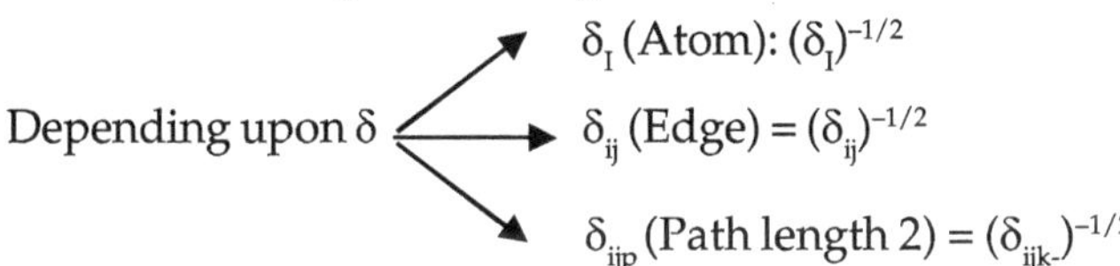

→ Zero-order, n = 0,

→ First-order, n = 1,

→ Second-order, n = 2, and

→ Third-order, n = 3

$^0\chi = 4.2845$ For

$^1\chi = 2.2700$

$^2\chi = 1.8022$

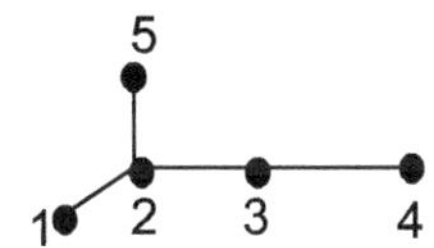

2.7.2. Extended Adjacency Matrix: EA

$E_A = \{g_{ij}\}$

$$\text{where, } g_{ij} = a_{ij} \frac{\frac{v_i}{v_j} + \frac{v_i}{v_i}}{2}$$

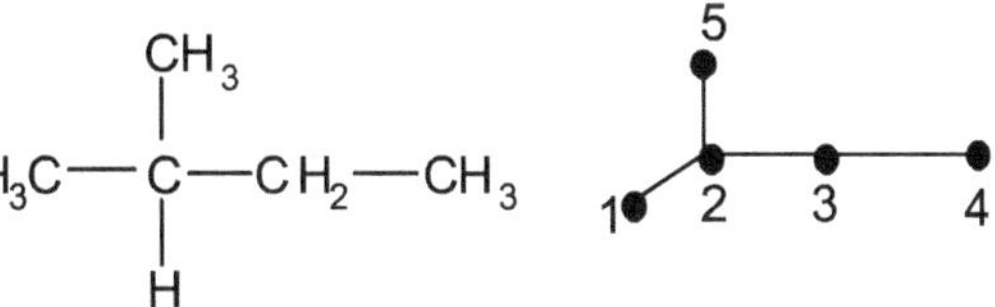

2-Methyl butane

It requires construction of adjacency matrix first.

		1	2	3	4	5	ΣV
	1	0	1	0	0	0	1
	2	1	0	1	1	0	3
A =	3	0	1	0	0	1	2
	4	0	0	1	0	0	1
	5	0	1	0	0	0	1
	ΣV	1	3	2	1	1	8

This gives degree vector = $V \equiv \{V_i\} = \{1\,3\,2\,1\,1\}$

∴ Extended adjacency matrix is constructed by calculating elements of EA matrix *i.e.*, g_{ij}.

Example

$$g_{21} = 1.\frac{\frac{3}{2}+\frac{1}{3}}{2} = 1.67$$

$$g_{32} = 1.\frac{\frac{2}{3}+\frac{3}{2}}{2} = 1.08, \ldots\ldots \text{ and so on.}$$

		1	2	3	4	5	ΣEA
	1	0	1.67	0	0	0	1.67
	2	1.67	0	1.08	1.67	0	4.42
EA =	3	0	1.08	0	0	1.25	2.33
	4	0	0	1.25	0	0	1.25
	5	0	1.67	0	0	0	1.67
	ΣEA	1.67	4.42	2.33	1.67	1.25	11.34

Sum of vertex vector of EA = 11.34

2.7.3. Distance Matrix (D)

(Discovered by Harary, 1969)

$$D_{ij} = \begin{cases} 1 & \text{if } i \neq j \\ 0 & \text{if } i = j \end{cases}$$

2-Methyl Butane

	1	2	3	4	5	ΣD_{ij}
1	0	1	2	3	2	8
2	1	0	1	2	1	5
3	2	1	0	1	2	6
4	3	2	1	0	3	9
5	2	1	2	3	0	8
ΣD_{ij}	8	5	6	9	8	36

Topological Indices Derived from D-matrix

(1) Wiener Index ≡ ½ Σ D_{ij}

(2) Polarity Number = P = ½ Σ entries of the order 3

(3) Plates Number = F = Σ Degrees of all edges

(4) Harary Index: H

(5) Balaban Index: J

≡ (a) Vertex Weighted.

(b) Edge Weighted.

(c) Vertex-Edge Weighted.

$$\text{Balaban Index (J)} \equiv \frac{M}{\mu+1}\sum(d_i d_j)^{-1/2}$$

where,

μ is the cyclometic number given by the following relationship:

μ = M – N + 1, Here, N is the number of non-hydrogen atoms.

M = 4 => Number of bonds
μ = 0 => Cyclomatic number

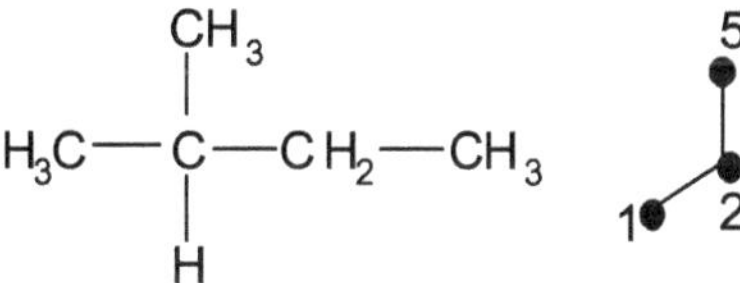

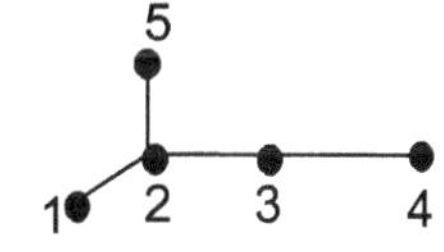

Minimum number of bonds required to convert cyclic compound into acyclic structure.

$\therefore$ J = $(8.5)^{-1/2} + (5.8)^{-1/2} + (5.6)^{-1/2} + (6.9)^{-1/2}$

= 2.5396

2.7.4. Bond Matrix

☆ Like Adjacency Matrix.

☆ Considers hydrogen contained graph.

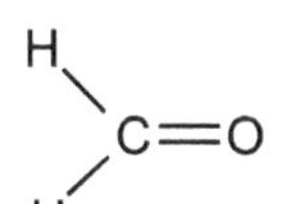

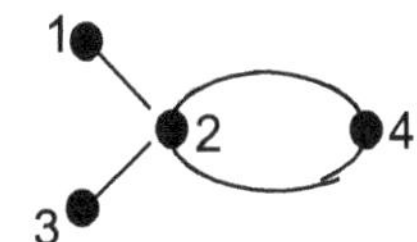

Example: Formaldehyde: HCHO ≡

	1	2	3	4	Σ
1	0	1	0	0	1
2	1	0	1	2	4
3	0	1	0	0	1
4	0	2	0	0	2
Σ	1	4	1	2	8

Σ = 1 + 4 + 1 + 2 = 8

2.7.5. Electron or Bond Electron Matrix

- ☆ Also called double booking bond matrix.
- ☆ Treatment is like adjacency matrix.
- ☆ Considers hydrogen contained graph.

Example: Formaldehyde: HCHO

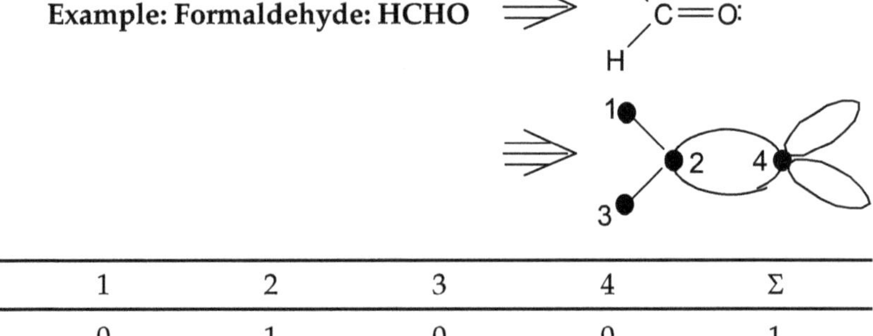

	1	2	3	4	Σ
1	0	1	0	0	1
2	1	0	1	2	4
3	0	1	0	0	1
4	0	2	0	4	6
Σ	1	4	1	6	12

$\Sigma = 1 + 4 + 1 + 6 = 12$

2.7.6. Detour Matrix (Δ)

- ☆ Maximum path matrix.

		1	2	3	4	5	6	Σ
	1	0	2	2	1	2	3	10
	2	2	0	2	3	4	1	12
Δ ≡	3	2	2	0	3	4	3	14
	4	1	3	3	0	1	4	12
	5	2	4	4	1	0	5	16
	6	3	1	3	4	5	0	16
	Σ	10	12	14	12	16	16	80

Δ Index = (80/2) = 40

2.7.7. Reciprocal Distance Matrix (D^{-1})

☆ $D^r_{ij} = 1/D_{ij}$ i ¹ J

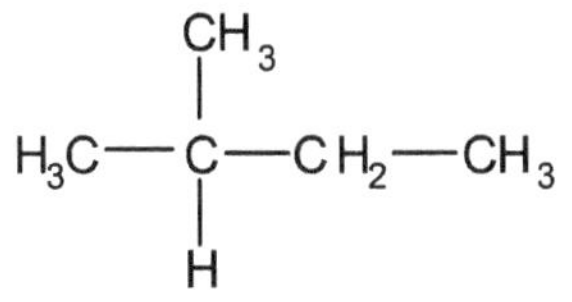

CH_3
H_3C—C—CH_2—CH_3
H

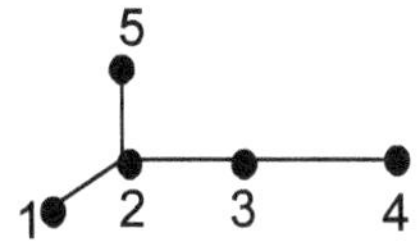

5
1 2 3 4

		1	2	3	4	5	Σ
	1	0	1	0.50	0.33	0.50	2.33
	2	1	0	1	0.50	1	3.50
$D^r \equiv$	3	0.50	1	0	1	0.50	3.00
	4	0.33	0.50	1	0	0.33	2.16
	5	0.50	1	0.50	0.33	0	2.33
	Σ	2.33	3.50	3.00	2.16	2.33	13.32

Harary Index H = ½ [2.33 + 3.50 + 3.00 + 2.16 + 2.33]
= ½ [13.32] = 6.66

2.7.8. Combinational Matrix: Schultz Matrix

V (A + B)   2-Methyl-butane

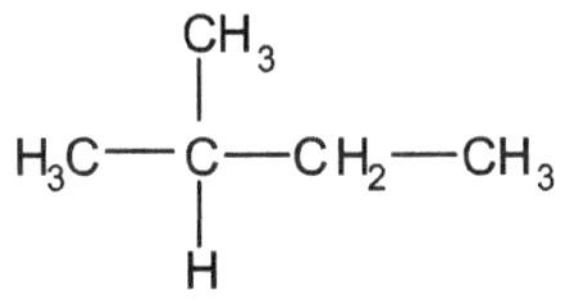

CH_3
H_3C—C—CH_2—CH_3
H

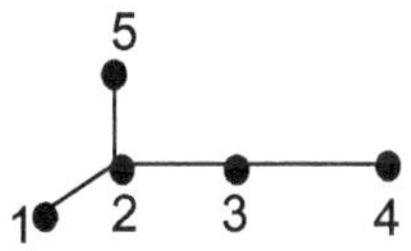

5
1 2 3 4

		1	2	3	4	5	Σ
	1	0	1	0	0	0	1
A =	2	1	0	1	0	1	3
	3	0	1	0	1	0	2
	4	0	0	1	0	0	1
	5	0	1	0	0	0	1
	Σ	1	3	2	1	1	8

V = Degree Vector ≡ { 1 3 2 1 1 }

		1	2	3	4	5
	1	0	1	2	3	2
	2	1	0	1	2	1
D ≡	3	2	1	0	1	2
	4	3	2	1	0	3
	5	2	1	2	3	0

		1	2	3	4	5
	1	0	2	2	3	2
	2	2	0	2	2	2
D+A ≡	3	2	2	0	2	2
	4	3	2	2	0	3
	5	2	2	2	3	0

$$V(D+A) \equiv \begin{bmatrix} 1 \\ 3 \\ 2 \\ 1 \\ 1 \end{bmatrix} \begin{bmatrix} 0 & 2 & 2 & 3 & 2 \\ 2 & 0 & 2 & 2 & 2 \\ 2 & 2 & 0 & 2 & 2 \\ 3 & 2 & 2 & 0 & 3 \\ 2 & 2 & 2 & 3 & 0 \end{bmatrix}$$

	0	2	2	3	2
	6	0	6	6	6
≡	4	4	0	4	4
	3	2	2	0	3
	2	2	2	3	0
	15	**10**	**12**	**16**	**15**

$\therefore V(D+A) = 68 = MTI$

2.7.9. Chemically Intuitive Adjacency Matrix

3-methyl-2-butanone: $CH_3COC_3H_7$

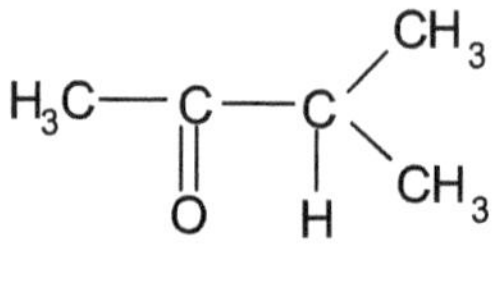

$$H_3C-\underset{\underset{O}{\|}}{C}-\underset{\underset{H}{|}}{C}\begin{matrix} CH_3 \\ CH_3 \end{matrix}$$

	C	H	H	H	C	O	C	H	C	H	H	H	C	H	H	H
C	0	1	1	1	1	0	0	0	0	0	0	0	0	0	0	0
H	1	0.15	0	0	0	0	0	0	0	0	0	0	0	0	0	0
H	1	0	0.15	0	0	0	0	0	0	0	0	0	0	0	0	0
H	1	0	0	0.15	0	0	0	0	0	0	0	0	0	0	0	0
C	1	0	0	0	0	√2	1	0	0	0	0	0	0	0	0	0
O	0	0	0	0	√2	0.9	0	0	0	0	0	0	0	0	0	0

C	0	0	0	0	1	0	0	1	1	0	0	0	1	0	0	0
H	0	0	0	0	0	0	1	0.15	0	0	0	0	0	0	0	0
C	0	0	0	0	0	0	1	0	0	1	1	1	0	0	0	0
H	0	0	0	0	0	0	0	0	1	0.15	0	0	0	0	0	0
H	0	0	0	0	0	0	0	0	1	0	0.15	0	0	0	0	0
H	0	0	0	0	0	0	0	0	1	0	0	0.15	0	0	0	0
C	0	0	0	0	0	0	1	0	0	0	0	0	0	1	1	1
H	0	0	0	0	0	0	0	0	0	0	0	0	1	0.15	0	0
H	0	0	0	0	0	0	0	0	0	0	0	0	1	0	0.15	0
H	0	0	0	0	0	0	0	0	0	0	0	0	1	0	0	0.15

The above Chemically Intuitive Molecular Index (CIMI) matrix is constructed using atomic parameters given below:

Atom	*Diagonal Element*
Carbon	0.00
Hydrogen	0.15
Nitrogen	0.90
Oxygen	0.90
Halogens	2.30

The eigen values of the above matrix is obtained as below and are then used as topological index.

λ_1	λ_2	λ_3	λ_4	λ_5	λ_6	λ_7	λ_8	λ_9	λ_{10}
2.380	2.362	2.292	2.069	1.809	1.659	1.537	0.849	0.781	0.638

It is worthy to record that:

(1) This modified adjacency matrix takes into account the electronic environment of the atoms so that the final eigen values have a strong empirical relationship to electron distribution of the molecule as a whole.

(2) The diagonal elements of the matrix need to reflect the electronic environment of a bonded, hybridized atom and this can be achieved by setting value of carbon to zero with non-zero values for other elements.

(3) These values are then adjusted to give a minimum in the standard error of prediction, SEP, of the data set.

(4) When the modified adjacency matrix is diagonalized to produce the eigen values it is important that the bonding electrons are included in proportion to their number.

(5) If the off-diagonal elements are thought to represent bonding electrons that are to be described, via the diagonalization algorithym, to the atoms, then they need to be encoded as the square-root of the bond-order, since perturbation theory shows that they will be added to the diagonal elements in proportion to the square of their value. This is achieved by setting the off-diagonal element representing bonding connections as 1, $\sqrt{2}$ and $\sqrt{3}$ for single, double and triple bonds respectively, where powers for bond order were investigated and were found to be less effective in practice. Other off-diagonal elements may be set to non-zero value to remove the likelihood of degeneracy as in the case of highly structural molecules or some isomeric structures.

(6) It might be thought that hydrogen atoms need only be included in the structures when the properties being modeled may be affected by their absence since their inclusion adds to the overheads of the diagonalization process.

2.8. Correlation Analysis[31-35]

Depending upon the structure one has to select an appropriate topological index for developing QSAR model. The recent trend in QSAR methodology is to select a large series of topological indices and then arrive at appropriate set of topological indices. This is done by correlation analysis, in that the set of topological indices are correlated with the biological activity of organic compounds acting as drugs. The correlation is then subjected to regression analysis employing the method of least squares. In regression analysis to show how representative of the results the correlation is, following parameters are used in correlation analysis:

(1) Number of compounds utilized (n),

(2) Correlation coefficient (r),

(3) Multiple correlation coefficient (R),

(4) Standard deviation (S),

(5) Standard error of estimation (Se), and

(6) Fisher's statistics (F).

2.8.1. Number of Compounds Utilized (n)

The quality of correlation depend upon the number of compounds utilized in the regression analysis. This number should be as high as possible. The value of r or R is then assessed with reference to n. The r or R varies in between –1 to +1 and the correlation is considered best, when r or R is nearer to –1 or +1.

2.8.2. Correlation Coefficient (r and R)

The correlation coefficient is expressed by r if it is simple correlation *i.e.*, involving only one parameter in regression analysis. If it is multiple correlation, *i.e.* involving two or more correlating parameters, correlation coefficient is expressed by R. High value of r or R > 0.90 indicates the statistical significance of the regression equation is high. The low value of r or R indicates that the correlation represented by the regression equation is least affected by the factor symbolised by that particular correlating parameter.

The linear regression (mono-parametric, one-variable, univariate) equation is represented by the following expression:

$$Y = mX + C \tag{2.13}$$

where,

X is the correlating parameter.

Or, $$BA = m\,IT + C \tag{2.14}$$

where,

BA is the biological activity, TI is topological index or any other correlating parameter, m is slope or coefficient of the correlating parameter and C is constant or intercept. X and Y represent variables, Y is dependent variable *i.e.* the drug activity under study and X is independent variable *i.e.* the correlating parameter. All these regression parameters are calculated using the following expression:

$$m = \frac{n.\sum XY - \sum X.\sum Y}{n\sum X^2 - (\sum X)^2} \tag{2.15}$$

The situation in multiparametric correlation is little bit different. The linear regression multiparameter dependent equation is written as –

$$C = \frac{\sum Y - m\sum X}{n} \tag{2.16}$$

$$r = \frac{n\sum XY - \sum X.\sum Y}{\sqrt{[n.\sum X^2 - (\sum X)^2][n.\sum Y^2 - (\sum Y)^2]}} \tag{2.17}$$

$$F = (n\text{-}1)\ \frac{r^2}{1-r} \tag{2.18}$$

$$t = r\sqrt{\frac{n-2}{1-r^2.m}} \tag{2.19}$$

$$S = \sqrt{\frac{\sum Y^2 - 2m\sum XY - 2c\sum Y + m^2\sum X^2 + 2mc\sum X + nc^2}{n-1}} \tag{2.20}$$

where,

$b_1, b_2, b_3, \ldots$ etc. are the coefficients to the corresponding correlating parameters $X_1, X_2, X_3, \ldots$ etc. and C is constant. For solving the above relationship, the following parameters are calculated. To make calculations more simple we consider two parametric correlation:

$$\log BA = b_1X_1 + X_2b_2 + c$$

for which we calculate,

$$D = (\Sigma X_1^2)(\Sigma X_2)^2 - (\Sigma X_1 X_2)^2 \quad (2.21)$$

$$b_2 = \frac{(\sum X_1^2)(\sum X_2)^2 - (\sum X_1X_2)(\sum X_1Y)}{D} \quad (2.22)$$

$$b_1 = \frac{(\sum X_2^2)(\sum X_1Y) - (\sum X_1Y)(\sum X_2Y)}{D} \quad (2.23)$$

$$F = \frac{\text{Regression SS}/2}{\text{Error SS}/n-3} \quad (2.24)$$

where,

Regression SS = Total SS – Error SS, (SS $\rightarrow$ Sum of squares)

$$\text{Total SS} = \sum_{i=1}^{n} (Y_i - \overline{Y})^2, \text{where, } \overline{Y} = \frac{\sum Y_i}{n}$$

$$= \sum Y_i^2 - n(\overline{Y})^2 \quad (2.24)$$

$$\text{Error SS} = \sum_{i=1}^{n} (Y_i - \hat{Y}_j)^2 \quad (2.25)$$

2.8.3. Standard Deviation (S)

The standard deviation (S) gives the idea about the precision of that regression expression. Greater the value of S, large will be the accuracy with which the expected value of the new compound may be guessed.

2.8.4. Coefficient of Variance (r^2)

This parameter explains about percent data represented by that particular regression expression. That is, if $r = 0.7$, then $r^2 = 0.49$ meaning thereby that 49 per cent data is accounted by regression of that parameter/s, still having 51 per cent data yet unaccounted. The value of r vis-à-vis r^2 can be improved by inclusion of another parameter. This term (r^2) helps us to understand whether other parameters should be sought for or not. Greater the value of r^2, lesser is the variance (data) that remains unaccounted by the regression equation.

2.8.5. Fisher Statistics (F)

The Fisher statistics (F) evaluates the statistical validity of a regression equation. For example, for 1 per cent probability level of statistical invalidity or insignificance, F = 13.74. Hence, for the regression equation if

F_{std} (*i.e.* 13.74) < $F_{calculated}$

Then the relationship represented by that equation is statistically significant.

2.9. Other Important Statistical Parameters

In addition to the above, the following important statistical parameters are sometimes used to explain the regression equation more precisely.

2.9.1. Poglaini Quality Parameter (Q)

The Poglaini quality parameter (Q) is expressed[36,37] as the ratio of correlation coefficient (R) to the standard error (S) *i.e.* Q = R/S and is used to decide predictive power of the derived regression equation. The larger the value of R, the smaller the S, the larger will be Q, and the better will be the predictive power of the derived regression equation.

2.9.2. Predictive Correlation Coefficient (r^2_{pred})

The predictive correlation coefficient (r^2_{pred}) is the another parameter[38,39] used to decide predictive power of the regression equation. This is obtained by correlating observed activity with the estimated activity, correlation coefficient of which gives r^2_{pred}.

2.9.3. Index of Forecasting Efficiency (E)[40]

$$E = 100\,[1 - \sqrt{(1 - r^2)}\,] \tag{2.27}$$

2.9.4. Coefficient of Alienation (k)[40]

$$k = \sqrt{(1 - r^2)} \tag{2.28}$$

2.9.5. Probable Error of Correlation Coefficient (PE)[40]

$$PE = \frac{2}{3}\,\frac{1 - r^2}{\sqrt{n}} \tag{2.29}$$

2.9.6. Goodness of Fit (SD)[40]

$$SD = \frac{\sqrt{\sum (\log obs - \log est)^2}}{n - 1 - k} \tag{2.30}$$

2.10. Achievements of QSAR

We now discuss the achievements of QSAR methodology and give them below:

(1) QSAR helps to understand the forces that given the activity in a congeneric series of compound.

(2) It helps to reduce the empiricism in drug-design and ensures that every drug synthesized and pharmacologically tested is as meaningful as possible.

(3) It helps forecasting of biological activity. The activity can be guessed from the regression process. However, QSAR is not the final answer to drug discovery. It may be considered as one of the refined tools for drug development.

(4) Selection of proper substituents or proper correlating parameters can be judged from the results of QSAR. It gives a good chance of finding combinations of parameters to optimise potency.

(5) With the introduction of QSAR the qualitative concept of bio-isosterism has turned to be more quantitative and constitutive. QSAR helps to decide an isoster which will give better pharmacokinetic and/or pharmacodynamic properties to the lead nucleus.

(6) The drug receptor interactives can be better understood by QSAR analysis. In a congeneric series of compounds, QSAR help to predict in quantitative terms, the forces involved in the drug receptor interactions. It is possible to derive a quantitative correlation between the strength of binding and the number and types bonds in drug-receptor interactions. If the selection of the parameter(s) is proper, QSAR may also suggest at which positions of the receptor, increased lipophilicity of drug increases binding, low changes in the strength of potential hydrogen bonds affect binding. The three dimensional feature of receptor and minimum energy active conformational forms of the drug molecules can also be predicted through QSAR analysis.

(7) Pharmacokinetic information can also be achieved from QSAR graphs. The correlation between variable types of parameters and the pharmacokinetic features of the drug can be done using QSAR. The passive reabsorption of substances from the urinary filtrate to decrease the total amount of drug, excreted in the urine can also be studied by QSAR analysis.

2.11. Limitations of QSAR

Even though the applications of QSAR analysis results into statistically valid equations, it is often difficult to interpret the relationship in biochemical terms. Failure of regression analysis in the prediction of biological activity of analogs results mainly due to the following:

(1) A poorly designed series or ambiguous regression analysis,

(2) An extrapolation outside the range of the physical properties represented by original correlating parameters,

(3) Improper conditions of the biological testing, and

(4) Multiple modes of action.

The most serious problem in QSAR is the lack of fundamental understanding of how to quantitatively descriple effects due to correlating parameters. Hence, the knowledge about the sort of interactions and quantification of correlating parameters effect on the interactions is essential.

A successful QSAR can provide only indirect information about the three dimensional aspects of drug-receptor interactions. However, mutual conformational adaptation of drug and receptor may also occur after interaction. Since no specific parameters has yet been developed for the description of the variation in conformation, conformational flexibility or three dimensional aspects of the drug, it imposes limitation on the success of QSAR analysis.

The electronic and steric parameters have their own influences on the overall lipophilicity of the molecule. This may result in the wrong correlation and interpretation of activity in a series that mainly depends upon lipophilicity for biological action. The electronic effect may change both the degree of ionization and the degree of distribution. The former may affect the amount of active species available to the receptor while the latter may affect the strength of the drug-receptor interaction. In addition, QSAR fails to explain scatter mathematically.

In the following Chapter III of the present thesis we describe the method of calculations of important topological indices commonly used in QSAR analysis.

References

1. Benigni, R., *Quantitative Structure-Activity Relationship (QSAR)*, Models of Mutagenes and Carcinogus, CRC Press: Bucaroton, FL 2003.
2. Diudea, M.V.; Ivancive, D., *Molecular Topology*, Complex, Cluj, 1995.
3. Diudea, M.V. (Ed.), *QSPR/QSAR Studies by Molecular Descriptors*, Nova Science, 2000.
4. Dericiers, J. (Ed.). *Comparative QSAR*, Taylor and Franes: Washington DC, 1998.
5. Kier, L.B.; Hall, L.H., *Molecular Structure Description. The Electro-topological State*, Academic: San Dieago, 1994.
6. Charton, M. (Ed.). *Advances in Quantitative Structure-Property Relationships*, Vol.1, JAI Press: Greenwich, 1996.
7. Balaban, A.J. (Ed.). *From Chemical Topology in Three-Dimensional Geometry*, Kluwer: Dordrecht, The Netherlands, 1997.
8. Cavallito, C.J. (Ed.). *Structure Activity Relationship*, Pergamon: New York, 1973.
9. Kier, L.B., *Molecular Orbital Theory in Drug Research*, Academic: New York, 1971.
10. Devillers, J. (Ed.). *Neural Networks in QSAR and Drug Design*, Academic Press, London, 1996.
11. Hansch, C.; Klein, T., *Acc. Chem. Res.*, **1986**, *19*, 392.
12. Hansch, C., *Acc. Chem. Res.*, **1993**, *26*, 147.
13. Pliska, V.; Testa, B.; Van de Waterbeemed (Eds.). *Lipophilicity in Drug Action and Toxicology*, VCH: Weinheim, 1996.

14. Estrada, E.; Patlewicz, G., *Croatica Chem. Acta*, **2004**, *77*, 203.
15. Todeschini, R.; Cunsonni, V., *Handbook of Molecular Descriptors*, Wiley, New York, 2001.
16. Karelson, M., *Molecular Descriptors in QSAR/QSPR*, Wiley: New York, 2000.
17. Devillies, J.; Balaban, A.T. (Eds.). *Topological Indices and Related Descriptors in QSAR and QSPR*, Taylor and Francis, 2000.
18. Kier, L.B.; Hall, L.H., *Molecular Structure Description*, Academic, London, 1999.
19. Bonohev, D., *Information Theoric Indices for Characterization of Chemical Structure*, Research Studies Press: Letchworn, 1983.
20. Zupan, J.; Gasteiger, J., *Neural Networks in Chemistry and Drug Design*, 2nd ed., Wiley, New York, 1999.
21. Hansch, C.; Kurup, A.; Garg, R.; Gao, H., *Chem. Rev.*, **2001**, *101*, 619.
22. Kubinyi, H., *QSAR: Hansch Analysis and Related Approaches*, VCH: Weinheim, 1994.
23. Hansch, C.; Fujita, J., ρ, σ, π Analysis, *J. Am. Chem. Soc.*, **1964**, *86*, 1616.
24. Hansch, C.; Leo, A., *Exploring QSAR Fundamentals and Applications in Chemistry and Biology*, American Chemical Society, Washington DC, 1995.
25. Hansch, C.; Leo, A.; Hoekman, D., *Exploring QSAR. Hydrophobic Electronic and Steric Constants*, American Chemical Society, Washington DC, 1995.
26. Free, S.M.; Wilson, J.W., *J. Med. Chem.*, **1964**, *7*, 395.
27. Free, S.M.; Wilson, J.W., Unpublished results.
28. Kubinyi, H.; Folkers, G.; Martin, Y.L. (Eds.), *3D QSAR in Drug Design: Recent Advances*, Kluwer/ESCOM, Amsterdam: The Netherlands, 1998.
29. Trinajstic, N., *Chemical Topology*, Vol.II, CRC Press, Boca Roton, FL, 1999.
30. Diudea, M.V.; Khadikar, P.V., *Molecular Topology and its Application*, Gilotia, New Delhi (In Press).
31. Chatterjee, S.; Hadi, A.S.; Price, B., *Regression Analysis by Examples*, 3rd ed., Wiley, New York, 2000.
32. DeMath, J.E., *Basic Statistics and Pharmaceutical Statistical Applications*, Marcel Dekker, New York, 1999.
33. Livingstone, D., *Data Analysis for Chemists, Applications to QSAR and Chemical Product Design*, Oxford University Press, 1995.
34. van de Waterbeemd (Ed.), *Chemonutric Methods in Molecular Design*, Vol.2, VCH Weinheim, 1995.
35. Senn, S., *Statistical Issues in Drug Development*, Wiley VCH, Weinheim, 1997.
36. Pogliani, L., *J. Phys. Chem.*, **1994**, *98*, 1494.
37. Pogliani, L., *Chem. Rev.*, **2000**, *100*, 3827.

38. Agrawal, V.K.; Bano, S.; Supuran, C.T.; Khadikar, P.V., *Eur. J. Med. Chem.*, **2004**, *39*, 593.

39. Agrawal, V.K.; Shrivastava, S.; Khadikar, P.V.; Supuran, C.T., *Bioorg. Med. Chem.*, **2003**, *11*, 5353.

40. Khadikar, P.V.; Singh, S.; Jaiswal, M.; Mandloi, D., *Bioorg. Med. Chem. Lett.*, **2004**, *14*, 4795.

Chapter 3

Topological Indices Commonly Used and Some Used in the Present Study

– Topological indices are useful tools for Quantitative Structure-Activity Relationship

– Alexendru T. Balaban, 1993

3.1. Introduction

In this Chapter III of the present thesis we describe the method of calculation of different types of topological indices which are more commonly used in QSAR analysis[1–3]. Out of these topological indices we have used Wiener (W)-[4], Szeged (Sz)-[5–7], Balaban (J)-[15,16], first-order molecular connectivity ($^1\chi$)-[11] and logRB[3] indices in the present study for modeling antibacterial activity of parent sulfa drugs together with those of Mannich bases derived from these sulfa drugs. In addition, these topological indices are also used in modeling anti-bacterial activity of Mannich bases derived from secondary amines.

The QSAR methodology presented in this thesis under "Results and Discussion" Chapter IV consists of the following:

(1) Modeling of antibacterial activity of Mannich bases on the basis of only carbon-hydrogen suppressed graph. All other heteroatom-hydrogen bonds are retained;

(2) Modeling of antibacterial activity of Mannich bases considering completely hydrogen-suppressed graph. That is, in these graphs all the carbon-hydrogen bonds alongwith heteroatom hydrogen bonds are deleted, and

(3) Modeling of antibacterial activity considering "rooted graph" of the Mannich bases. In this methodology the molecular graph is rooted at the substituent R and, therefore, corresponds to molecular graph of the 'substituents'.

Consequently, the results obtained using type (2) of graphs corresponds to global structure of the molecule, while the results obtained from the rooted graphs are used to discuss effect of the antibacterial activity of the Mannich bases due to substitution. That is, it reflects substitution effect.

As stated in Chapter II of the present thesis, the calculations of the topological indices is done using completely suppressed molecular graphs. The calculations of important topological indices are given below:

3.1.1. Wiener Index (W)

The Wiener index (W)[4] of a graph G is just the sum of distances of all pairs of vertices of G:

$$W = W(G) = \tfrac{1}{2}\Sigma d(v, \mu \mid G) \tag{3.1}$$

where,

d(v | G) is called the distance number (minimum distances of vertex v and is defined as:

$$d(V \mid G) = \sum_{\mu \in V(G)} d(v, \mu \mid G) \tag{3.2}$$

3.1.2. Szeged Index (Sz)[5-7]

The Szeged index (Sz) of a graph G is defined as:

$$Sz = Sz(G) = \sum_{e \in E(G)} [n_1(e \mid G)\, n_2(e \mid G)] \tag{3.3}$$

where,

$n_1(e \mid G)$ and $n_2(e \mid G)$ count the vertices of G close to the vertices u and v, respectively. The vertices equidistant from both the ends of an edge are not taken into account.

3.1.3. PI (Padmakar-Ivan) Index (PI)[8-10]

The PI (Padmakar-Ivan) index, PI = PI(G) of the graph G is defined as:

$$PI = PI(G) = \sum_{e \in E(G)} [n_{eu}(e \mid G) + n_{ev}(e \mid G)] \tag{3.4}$$

where,

n_{eu} and n_{ev} are the number of edges nearer to u and v of the two ends of the edge e = uv. Like Szeged index (Sz) here also the edges equidistant from the two ends of the edge are not counted in the calculation of PI index.

3.1.4. Randic Indices ($^0\chi$, $^1\chi$ and $^2\chi$)

The Randic index $^1\chi = {}^1\chi(G)$ of G was introduced by Randic in 1975 as the connectivity index[11]. This index is one of the most widely used topological indices in QSPR/QSAR analyses. In its original form it is defined as below:

$$^1\chi = {}^1\chi(G) = \sum_{ij} [\delta_i \delta_j]^{-1/2} \tag{3.5}$$

where,

δ_i is the valence of a vertex i, equal to the number of bonds connected to the atom i, in G, representing the graph of a compound. The meaning of δ_j is analogous. The expressions for computing $^0\chi$ and $^2\chi$ are analogous.

3.1.5. Kier and Hall Valence Connectivity Indices ($^0\chi^v$, $^1\chi^v$ and $^2\chi^v$)

In an attempt to include multiple bonds and heteroatoms in the Randic index[11], Kier and Hall[12–14] proposed the alence values of atoms according to the following equation

$$\delta_i^v = Z^v - h_i \tag{3.6}$$

where,

Z^v is the number of valence electrons of atom i and h_I is the number of hydrogens bonded to it. Thus, the Randic connectivity index was modified by Kier and Hall replacing δ_i with δ_I^v.

The Randic/Kier/Hall approach has been applied successfully to a variety of physicochemical and biological activities.

3.1.6. Balaban Index (J)

The Balaban index[15,16] J = J(G), was introduced by Balaban in 1982 as the average distance sum connectivity index. It is defined as –

$$J = \frac{M}{\mu+1} \sum_{\text{all edges}} (d_i d_j)^{-0.5} \tag{3.7}$$

where,

M is the number of edges of G, μ is the cyclomatic number of G; and d_i is the distance sum, where i = 1,2,3…,n. The cyclomatic number equals the minimum number of edges that must be removed from G in order to transform it to the related acyclic graph. Alternatively μ is calculated using the following relationship:

$$\mu = M - N + 1$$

where,

N is the number of non-hydrogen atoms in the graph G.

3.1.7. Balaban Heteroatom Index (J_{HET})[15]

This is an extension of Balaban index (J) to molecules containing heteroatoms. In the case of heteroatoms differentiation is made between the atoms of different kinds by modifying the corresponding elements of the distance matrix D. For instance, the following modification was suggested for the diagonal elements.

$$(D)_{ij} = 1 - (Z_c/Z_i) \quad (3.8)$$

where,

$Z_c = 6$ and Z_i is determined by the number of all electrons of atom i or namely Z_i is the atomic number of given elements.

The off-diagonal elements of the modified distance matrix for heteroatom systems are given by the following equation.

$$(D)_{ij} = \sum_{r} k_r \quad (3.9)$$

where,

the summation is over r bonds.

The bond parameter k_r is given by the following expression.

$$k_r = 1/w_r X(Z_c)^2/(Z_i+Z_j) \quad (3.10)$$

where,

w_r is the bond weight with values of 1, 1.5, 2 and 3 for a single, aromatic, double, and triple bond, respectively.

3.1.8. Schultz Index (MTI)[17]

The Schultz index, MTI = MTI (G) of G, was introduced by Schultz in 1989 as the molecular topological index and is defined by the following expression:

$$\text{MTI} = \sum_{i=1}^{N} e_i \quad (3.11)$$

where,

e_i (i = 1,2,3,....,N) represents the elements of the row matrix of order N.

$$V(A+D) = (e_1\, e_2\, e_3 \ldots N) \quad (3.12)$$

where,

V is the valence row matrix, A is the adjacency matrix and D is the distance matrix.

3.1.9. Harary Index (H)

The Harary index[18–21], H = H(G) of G, was introduced by Plasvic *et al.*, in 1991 in honour of Prof. Frank Harary on his 70th birth day. It is defined as –

$$H = ½ \sum_{i=1}^{N} \sum_{i=j}^{N} (D_{ij})^{-2} \quad (3.13)$$

where,

D^{-2} is the matrix whose elements are the squares of the reciprocal distances in G.

3.1.10. Extended Adjacency Indices (EAΣ and EA_{max})

The extended adjacency matrix indices[22,23] EAΣ and EA_{max} were introduced by Yang *et al.*, in 1994. These indices are based on the extended adjacency matrices of molecules in that they influence factors of heteroatoms and multiple bonds which were considered. These indices possesses high discriminating power and correlate with a number of physicochemical properties and biological activities of organic compounds. They are defined as –

$$EA = \{g_{ij}\} \tag{3.14}$$

where,

$g_{ij} = a_{ij}\,[(v_i/v_j) + (v_j/v_i)]/2$ are the elements of the EA matrix and a_{ij} denotes elements of the A matrix.

EAΣ is the sum of the absolute eigen values of the EA matrix, and EA_{max} is the maximum of the absolute eigen values of the EA matrix.

3.1.11. Zagreb Group Indices (M_1 and M_2)[24]

These indices are based on π-electron energy, in which two terms appear in the approximate formula for the total π-energy which are used separately as topological indices. They are defined as

$$M_1(G) = \sum_{j=1}^{N} D_j^2 \tag{3.15}$$

$$M_2(G) = \sum_{ij}^{N} D_j D_j \tag{3.16}$$

The symbol D_i stands for the valency of the vertex i. The sum over in eq.() is over all vertices of G, while the sum in eq.() is over all edges.

3.1.12. Information Indices (I)

Bonchev and Trinajstic[24] applied information theory to the problem of characterizing molecular structure. The information content of the system i with N elements is defined by the following relationship:

$$I = N \log_2 N - \sum_{j=1}^{n} N_j \log_2 N_j \tag{3.17}$$

where,

n is the number of different sets of elements, $N\text{-}_j$ is the number of elements in the jth set of elements, and summation is over all sets of elements. The logarithm is taken at the base 2 for measuring information contents in bytes.

3.1.13. Topological I-Index

Topological I-index[25] of a graph G is based on the topological distances from a given vertex in the edge weighted graph of the organic molecule and is defined as –

$$I = \frac{\sum_{r=1}^{N} n_r g_r}{\sum_{j=1}^{N} n_r} \tag{3.18}$$

where,

n_r is the number of rth kind of vertices for which g_r is the topological distance from the root in the edge weighted graph and the topological distance d_{ij} between the vertices I and j is defined as the distance associated with a minimum weight. The weights in the edge-weighted graphs correspond to k values of the Huckel parameter[26,27] for the heteroatom.

3.1.14. Path Numbers (P_n) as Molecular Descriptors (Atomic I_D number)

Path numbers[28,29] have been used as molecular descriptors to compare structures. Paths or self-avoiding walks are enumerated first for individual atoms in a structure – this yields the atomic path sequence a_1, a_2, a_3,....,a_n. The first number gives the number of paths of length one for a considered atom. Next is the number of paths of length two and so on.

If path numbers for all atoms are added (and divided by two, since each path involves two atoms as terminate), one obtains a path sequence for a molecule as a whole: m_1, m_2,...., m_n. Such a sequence can be preceded by m_0, the number of atoms in a molecule (graph).

If paths (weighted or otherwise) for each atom are added, one obtains a single number representation of each atom (vertex) in a graph g; such atomic parameters are called an atomic identification number or an atomic I_D number[30,31] and be used in QSPR/QSDAR studies.

3.1.15. Molecular I_D Number

Similar to an atomic I_D number[32,33] is the molecular I_D number defined as the sum of all paths (weighted or nonweighted) in a molecule (graph). This index carries considerable structural information and is successfully used in QSPR/QSAR analyses.

3.1.16. Mean Wiener Index[30,34] (W_m)

The mean value of topological distances is defined[35,36] as –

$$W_m = W_m(G) = \{I/N(N-1)\} \sum_{ij} d_{ij} \tag{3.19}$$

where, n is the number of vertices (atoms). The summation is taken over all the elements of distance matrix, D.

The total number of elements in a triangular off-diagonal submatrix is equal to ½{N(N-1)}. Therefore, the mean Wiener index (mean value of the Wiener number) is given by the following expression

$$W_m(G) = 2W/N(N-1) \quad (3.20)$$

3.1.17. Mean Square Wiener Index (W_{ms})

The mean square value of the Wiener number is defined[30,36,39] as the mean of the square of the elements of the off-diagonal submatrix.

$$W_{ms} = W_{ms}(G) = \{1/N(N-1)\} \sum_{ij} d_{ij}^2 \quad (3.21)$$

3.1.18. Root-Mean-Square Wiener Index (W_{rms})

The root-mean-square value of the Wiener number[38] is defined as the square root of the mean of the square of the elements of the off-diagonal submatrix:

$$W_{rms} = W_{rms}(G) = [\{1/N(N-1)\}] \sum_{ij} d_{ij}^2{}_{0.5} \quad (3.22)$$

Trinajstic[24] while disucssing topological indices and their applications to structure-property and structure-activity relationships recommended that the Randic connectivity index[11] is the most used topological index, and this index and its variants be used in QSPR/QSAR studies at a priority level. Also that the information index, though complicated, can also be used easily for QSAR studies. Finally, the recommended that the Balaban index[15] (J and J_{HET}) has favourable features for use in QSPR/QSAR studies and stated that preliminary results in this direction are promising.

References

1. Devillers, J., *Comparative QSAR*, Taylor and Francis, Philadelphia, 1998.
2. Trinajstic, N., *Chemical Graph Theory*, 2nd ed., CRC Press, Boca Raton, Florida, 1992.
3. Kier, L.B. and Hall, L.H., *Molecular Structure Description*, Academic Press, New York, 1999.
4. Wiener, H., *J. Am. Chem. Soc.*, **1947**, *69*, 17.
5. Gutman, I., *Graph Theory Notes*, New York, **1994**, *27*, 9.
6. Khadikar, P.V., Deshpande, N.V., Kale, P.P., Dobrynin, A., Gutman, I. and Domotor, G., *J. Chem. Inf. Comput. Sci.*, **1995**, *35*, 547.
7. Khadikar, P.V., Mandloi, D. and Bajaj, A.V., *Oxid. Commun.*, **2004**, *27*, 23.
8. Khadikar, P.V., *Nat. Acad. Sci. Lett.*, **2000**, *23*, 113.

9. Khadikar, P.V., Karmarkar, S. and Agrawal, V., *J. Chem. Inf. Comput. Sci.*, **2001**, *41*, 934.

10. Khadikar, P.V., Kale, P.P., Deshpande, N.V., Karmarkar, S. and Agrawal, V.K., *J. Math. Chem.*, **2001**, *29*, 143.

11. Randic, M., *J. Am. Chem. Soc.*, **1975**, *97*, 6609.

12. Kier, L.B., Hall, L.H., *Molecular Connectivity in Structure-Activity Relationship*, Wiley, New York, 1986.

13. Kier, L.B., Hall, L.H., *Molecular Connectivity in Chemistry and Drug Research*, Academic Press, New York, 1976.

14. Kier, L.B., Hall, L.H., Recent advances in molecular connectivity for biological SAR analysis. In *IUPAC Pesticide Chemistry Human Welfare and the Environment*, Miyamoto, J., Ed., Pergamon Press: 1983, 351.

15. Balaban, A.T., *Chem. Phys. Lett.*, **1982**, *89*, 399-404.

16. Balaban, A.T., *Theor. Chim. Acta*, **1979**, *53*, 355-375.

17. Schultz, H.P., *J. Chem. Inf. Comput. Sci.*, **1989**, *29*, 227-228.

18. Plavsic, D., Nicolic, S., Trinajstic, N., Mihalic, Z., *J. Math. Chem.*, **1993**, *12*, 235-250.

19. Mihalic, Z., Trinajstic, N., *J. Chem. Educ.*, **1992**, 609, 701-712.

20. Joshi, S., Singh, S., Agrawal, V.K., Mathur, K.C., Karmarkar, S., Khadikar, P.V., *Nat. Acad. Sci. Lett.*, **1999**, 22, 159-167.

21. Karmarkar, S., Thukral, G.S., Agrawal, V.K., Mathur, K.C., Khadikar, P.V., *Nat. Acad. Sci. Lett.*, **1999**, 22, 207-211.

22. Yang, Yi-Qiu, Xu, Lu., Hu Chang-Yu., *J. Chem. Inf. Comput. Sci.*, **1994**, *34*, 1140-1145.

23. Yao, Yu-Yuan, Xu, Lu., Yang, Yi-Qiu, Yuan Xiu-Shun., *J. Chem. Inf. Comput. Sci.*, **1993**, *33*, 590-594.

24. Trinajstic, N., *Chemical Graph Theory*, CRC Press, Boca Raton, FL, 1983, Voo.II, Chapter IV.

25. Lall, R.S., *Asian J. Chem.*, **1990**, *2*, 37-42.

26. Baryz, M., Jashari, G., Lall, R.S., Srivastava, Y.K., Trinajstic, N., In *Chemical Applications of Topology and Graph Theory*, King, R.b., Ed., Elsevier, Amsterdam, 1983, pp. 222-230.

27. Streitwieser, A., Jr. *Molecular Orbital Theory for Organic Chemists*, Wiley, New York, 1961.

28. Platt, J.R., *J. Chem. Phys.*, **1947**, *15*, 419-420.

29. Randic, M., *J. Math. Chem.*, **1992**, *9*, 97-146.

30. Randic, M., Jerman-Blazic, B., Grossman, S.C., Rouvary, D.H., *Math. Comput. Modelling*, **1988**, *9*, 571-582.

31. Randic, M., Jerman-Blazic, B., Rouvary, D.H. Seybold, P.G., Grossman, S.C., *Int. J. Quantum Chem., Quantum Biol. Symp.*, **1987**, *14*, 245-260.

32. Randic, M., *J. Chem. Inf. Comput. Sci.*, **1984**, *24*, 164-175.

33. Carter, S., Trinajstic, N., Nikolic, S., *Med. Sci. Res.*, **1988**, *16*, 185-186.

34. Karmarkar, S., Khadikar, P.V., Agrawal, V.K., Mathur, K.C., Mandloi, M., Joshi, S., *Proc. Indian acad. Sci. (Chem. Sec.)*, **2000**, *112*, 43-49.

35. Lall, R.S., *Current Sci.*, **1981**, *50*, 668-670.

36. Lall, R.S., *Indian J. Biochem. Biophys.*, **1988**, *25*, 364-367.

37. Khadikar, P.V., Joshi, S., *X-ray Spectro.*, **1995**, *24*, 201-204.

38. Mathur, K.C., Singh, S., Mathur, S., Khadikar, P.V., *Poll. Res.*, **1999**, *18*, 405-409.

Chapter 4
Results and Discussion

– We all have to learn that not all researches can result in publishable outcomes. Such things happened before and will appear in future too.

– Ivan Gutman, 1995

4.1. QSAR Study on the Antibacterial Activity of some Sulfa Drugs: Building Blockers of Mannich Bases

4.1.1. Introduction

The importance of sulfa drugs (sulfonamides) is well established in pharmaceutical chemistry and drug design. This class of drugs are well known as anti-bacterial, carbonic anhydrase inhibitors, anti-cancerous and also as anti-inflammatory agents. Consequent to these physiological activities of sulfa drugs they are used as building blockers for making Mannich bases[1,2].

In our earlier studies[3–16] several Mannich bases were synthesized from the sulfa drugs and have evaluated for their biological significance and toxicity, in particular anti-bacterial activity. However, to understand the biological potential of the derived Mannich bases, the same should be known for their building blockers *e.g.*, sulfa drugs. This can be done more efficiently by investigating Quantitative Structure-Activity Relationship (QSAR) study using distance-based topological indices[17–21]. Such a study for the sulfa drugs used in the present study (Table 4.1.1) are not reported in the literature. Thus, the present work deals with the antibacterial activity of sulfa drugs (Table 4.1.1) against *E. coli, K. pneumonae,* and *B. subtilis.* In doing so we have used distance-based topological indices: Wiener (W)[17]; Szeged index (Sz)[20,21], first-order connectivity index ($^1\chi$)[18] and Balaban index (J)[19]. The details of these indices are given in the chapter II and III of the present thesis.

Table 4.1.1: Molecular Structures of the Sulfa Drugs Used in the Present Study

1. **Sulfadiazine**

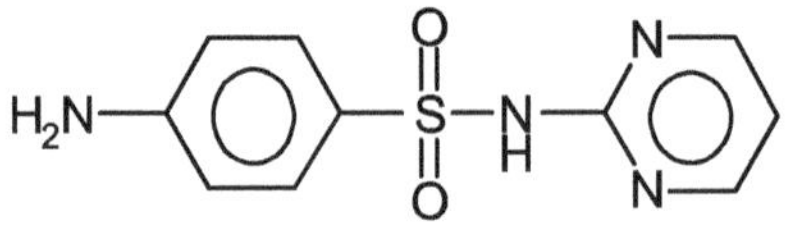

2. **Sulfamethoxazole**

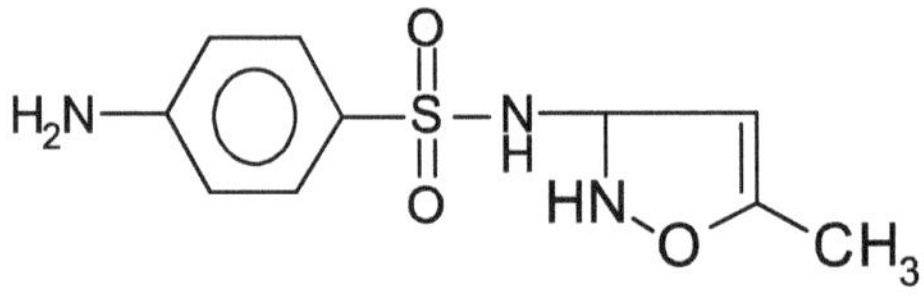

3. **Sulfaguanidine**

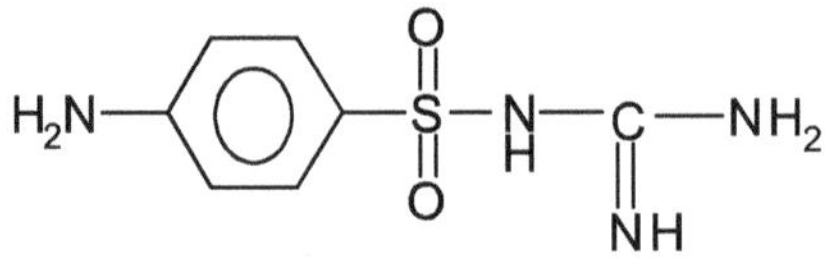

4. **Sulfadimidine**

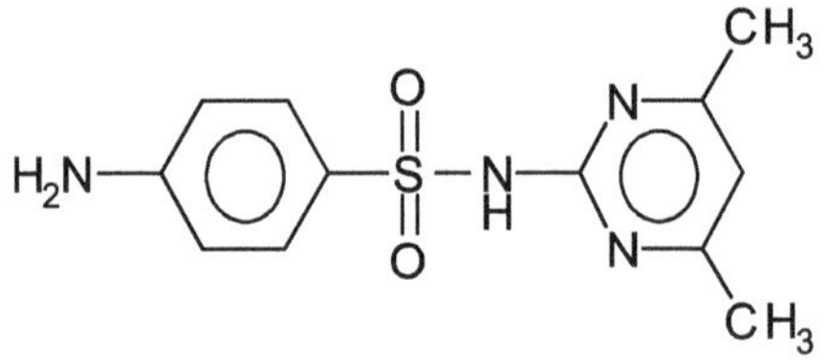

5. **Sulfamethiazole**

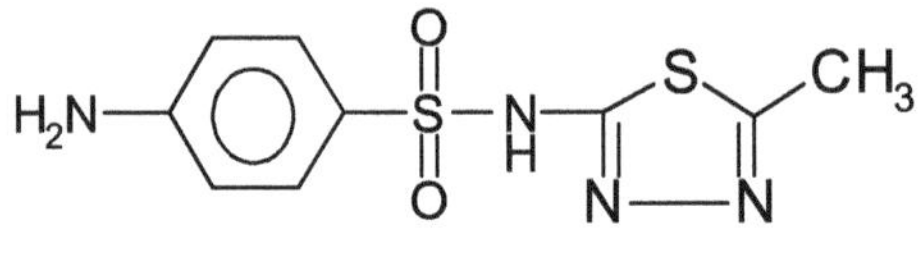

6. **Sulfanilamide**

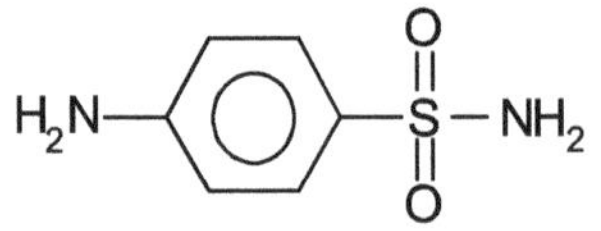

Before discussing the results obtained in the present study, it is worthy to mention that QSAR methodology is very useful in screening a large library of possible drug candidates for selectivity and potency[22–27]. Mathematical models are formed that correlate molecular structure to an activity or property of interest. Molecular structure is encoded through the generation of descriptors, which are numerical values corresponding to topological, geometric, or electronic structural features. The goal of

QSAR methodology is to develop several models to predict activity/property/toxicity using correlation analysis employing statistical techniques. In the present study we have used simple as well as multiple regression analysis using maximum R^2 methods[28].

4.1.2. Results and Discussion

The molecular structures of sulfa drugs used in the present study are given in Table 4.1.1 and their anti-bacterial activities against *E. coli, K. pneumonae* and *B. subtilis* are present in Table 4.1.2. The calculated values of distance-based topological indices: W, Sz, $^1\chi$, J, logRB are summarized in Table 4.1.3.

Table 4.1.2: Anti-bacterial Activity of the Sulfa Drugs against *E. coli, K. pneumonae* and *B. subtilis*

Sl.No.	Compound	Zone of Inhibition in mm				
		Concentration in µg/ml				Average
		10	20	40	80	
E. coli						
1.	1	9.70	17.20	21.20	24.50	18.14
2.	2	19.63	22.93	23.23	24.03	22.45
3.	4	15.10	16.90	18.80	18.56	17.34
4.	5	16.20	17.43	22.20	25.50	20.32
5.	6	20.43	22.30	22.86	25.55	22.78
K. pneumonae						
1.	1	27.03	29.23	29.53	25.63	27.83
2.	2	11.63	14.92	22.43	26.46	18.86
3.	5	30.33	29.86	29.60	27.76	29.39
B. subtilis						
1.	1	20.86	27.23	26.36	25.93	25.10
2.	2	22.80	25.46	27.43	27.90	25.90
3.	3	11.23	10.90	17.90	21.76	15.45
4.	4	15.40	19.96	21.76	22.08	19.80
5.	5	18.06	19.13	19.46	20.50	19.29

A perusal of Table 4.1.2 shows that only five sulfa drugs are effective against *E. coli*, however, against *K. pneumonae* only three *viz.*, 1, 2 and 5 are effective. In case of *B. Subtilis* sulfa drug no.6 is not effective. In obtaining QSAR models we have used average value of zone of inhibition to account for their anti-bacterial activities against the three bacteria mentioned earlier. Based on these average values we obtained the following order of antibacterial activity:

Against E. coli

$$6 > 2 > 5 > 1 > 4 \tag{4.1.1}$$

Against K. pneumonae

$$5 > 1 > 2 \tag{4.1.2}$$

Against B. subtilis

$$2 > 1 > 4 > 5 > 3 \tag{4.1.3}$$

Table 4.1.3: Distance Based Topological Indices Calculated for Sulfa Drugs Used in the Present Study

Sl.No.	Compound	Topological Indices				
		W	Sz	$^1\chi$	J	logRB
1.	1	536	818	8.0773	1.8372	162.0572
2.	2	535	731	7.9712	1.8479	161.6517
3.	3	307	427	6.4155	2.4613	96.2437
4.	4	722	1092	8.8650	1.8868	215.2262
5.	5	535	731	7.9712	1.8479	161.6517
6.	6	152	236	4.9990	2.3936	48.2757

It is interesting to record that only sulfa drug no.3 is active only against *B. subtilis* and it is inactive against other two bacteria. Furthermore, these sequences (order) do not establish any quantitative structure-activity (QSAR) relationship. Therefore, we have made such study using topological indices which encodes the molecular structures of sulfa drugs numerically. Since, different sulfa drugs are found effective against the three bacteria used we have obtained three different correlation matrices (Table 4.1.4) for preliminary investigation of correlatedness of topological indices against the anti-bacterial activity and also for investigating mutual correlatedness among the topological indices used. We will divide our discussion in the following three different headings based on the bacteria used.

4.1.2.1. Antibacterial Activity of Sulfa Drugs against *E. coli*

The data presented in Table 4.1.4 show that the topological indices W, Sz, $^1\chi$ and log RB are significantly correlated with the antibacterial activity against *E. coli* and that Sz is the best topological index for this purpose. The correlation potential of Balaban index (J) is significantly lower than the other topological indices. This shows that we can obtained four mono-parametric models for modeling antibacterial activity against *E. coli* and that mono-parametric model based on Sz will be the best for this purpose. This Table 4.1.4 also shows that all the five topological indices are highly linearly correlated and thus any combination of these indices in multilinear regression analysis may result with a model suffering from the defect due to collinearity. However, such cases are nicely dealt with by Randic[29] and we will follow his recommendation to explain model containing highly correlated topological indices. Looking to the sample size and following "Rule of Thumb" we can at the most go for bi-parametric regression analysis.

Table 4.1.4: Correlation Matrices for the Sulfa Drugs Used

	Activity	*W*	*Sz*	$^1\chi$	*J*	*logRB*
E. coli (n = 5)						
Activity	1.0000					
W	–0.74316	1.0000				
Sz	–0.81869	0.98966	1.0000			
$^1\chi$	–0.71278	0.98908	0.96911	1.0000		
J	0.55374	–0.88960	–0.84188	–0.94645	1.0000	
logRB	–0.74081	0.99994	0.98875	0.99058	–0.89442	1.0000
K. pneumonae (n = 3)						
Activity	1.0000					
W	0.37815	1.0000				
Sz	0.37815	1.0000	1.0000			
$^1\chi$	0.37815	1.0000	1.0000	1.0000		
J	–0.37815	–1.0000	–1.0000	–1.0000	1.0000	
logRB	0.37815	1.0000	1.0000	1.0000	–1.0000	1.0000
B. subtilis (n = 5)						
Activity	1.0000					
W	0.40917	1.0000				
Sz	0.38494	0.98630	1.0000			
$^1\chi$	0.51942	0.98772	0.96965	1.0000		
J	–0.75239	–0.79654	–0.74201	–0.87764	1.0000	
logRB	0.41002	1.0000	0.98647	0.98790	–0.79698	1.0000

The regression parameters and quality of correlation for the different mono- and bi-parametric models are given in Table 4.1.5. This shows that among the mono-parametric models, the model based on Sz gives better results:

Anti-bacterial activity against *E. coli* = 24.9010 – 0.0065 (± 0.0026) Sz (4.1.4)

n = 5, Se = 1.6295, r = -0.8187, F = 6.0980, Q = 0.5024

Here and thereafter n - is the number of compounds, Se – standard error of estimation, r – simple correlation coefficient, F – Fisher's statistics, and Q – quality factor, which is defined[29–34] as the ratio of correlation coefficient to the standard error of estimation *i.e.*, Q = r/Se).

The coefficient of Sz in the mono-parametric model represented by [eqn.(4.1.1)] is negative indicating thereby that anti-bacterial activity of sulfa drugs against *E. coli* is inversely proportional to the magnitude of Sz. This index Sz precisely accounts for the cyclic nature of the compound, whose negative coefficient in [eqn. (4.1.1)] indicates that the activity decreases with the increase in number of cycles present in the sulfa drugs.

As stated earlier we have attempted several bi-parametric regressions and the results obtained are presented in Table 4.1.5. These results show that the bi-parametric model containing W and Sz gave excellent results in accordance with the following expression:

Anti-bacterial activity against *E. coli* = 24.3154 + 0.0384 (± 0.0194) W - 0.0321 (± 0.0131) Sz (4.1.5)

$n = 5, Se = 1.1584, r = 0.9428, R^2_A = 0.7778, F = 8.001, Q = 0.8139$

Table 4.1.5: Regression Analysis and Quality of Correlation for Modeling Antibacterial Activity of Sulfa Drugs against *E. coli*

Model	*TI*	*Se*	R^2_A	*R*	*F*	*Q*
1	W	1.8987	–	–0.7432	3.701	0.3914
2.	Sz	1.6295	–	–0.8187	6.098	0.5024
3.	$^1\chi$	1.9903	–	–0.7128	3.098	0.3581
4.	J	2.3629	–	0.5537	1.327	0.2343
5.	logRB	1.9061	–	–0.7408	3.649	0.3886
6.	W, J	2.1772	0.2151	0.7795	1.548	0.3580
7.	Sz, J	1.7948	0.4666	0.8563	2.750	0.4771
8.	$^1\chi$, J	2.0613	0.2964	0.8051	1.843	0.3906
9.	J, logRB	2.1758	0.2161	0.7798	1.551	0.3584
10.	W, Sz	1.1584	0.7778	0.9428	8.001	0.8139
11.	W, $^1\chi$	2.2654	0.1502	0.7584	1.354	0.3347
12.	Sz, $^1\chi$	1.6408	0.5542	0.8815	3.487	0.5372

The physical significance of the negative coefficient of Sz term in the [eqn. (4.1.5)] is the same as discussed for [eqn. (4.1.4)]. The positive coefficient of W indicates that tree-like (acyclic) side chain is favourable for the exhibition of anti-bacterial activity of sulfonamides against *E. coli.* This bi-parametric model though violets "Rule of Thumb" and be considered statistically good as the coefficients of W and Sz are larger than their standard deviation. Furthermore, bi-parametric model [eqn.(4.1.5)] contains two highly linearly correlated topological indices, *viz.*, W and Sz and, therefore, needs further explanation. The multi-collinearity (auto-correlation) occurs when two independent variables are correlated with each other and this problem continue to be of prime concern to theoretical statistician. From a decision makers view point, one has to recognize the following problems and indication of severe multicollinearity:

(1) Incorrect signs of the coefficients,

(2) A change in the values of the previous coefficient, when a new variable is added for the model,

(3) Change to insignificant of a previously significant variable when a new variable is added to the model, and

(4) An increase in the standard error of the estimate when a variable is added to the model.

In addition, decision makers should also consider the recommendations of Randic[29], who stated that selection of descriptors to be used in QSAR studies should not be delegated solely to the computers, although the statistical criteria will continue to be useful for preliminary screening of the descriptors taken from a large pool. Often in a automated selection of descriptors a descriptor will be discarded because it is highly correlated with another descriptor already selected, what is more important is not descriptor parallel to one another, but whether they differ in those parts that are important to QSAR correlations. If they differ in the domain, which is important for the QSAR both descriptors should be retained. If they differ in parts that are not relevant for the correlation, one of them can be discarded. Thus, we observed that none of the four problems/indications of multi-collinearity are present in the model expressed by [eqn. (4.1.5)]. Also that both W and Sz indices carry different information content. The W index basically accounts for effect due to acyclic side-chain (tree-like structure), while Sz index deals primarily with cyclic nature of the molecule. Hence, the model [eqn. (4.1.1)] though not very good for theoretical statistician, it is excellent from chemical point of view. The coefficients of both W and Sz terms are significantly larger than their respective standard deviation, further supporting that model [eqn.(4.1.1)] is an excellent model for monitoring, modeling and estimating antibacterial activity of sulfa drugs against *E. coli.*

In order to confirm our results we have estimated the antibacterial activity of sulfa drugs against *E. coli* using model expressed by [eqn.(4.1.5)] and compared them with the observed values. The data presented in Table 4.1.6 show that the observed and the estimated activities are very close to each other.

Table 4.1.6: Found and Estimated Antibacterial Activity of Sulfa Drug against *E. coli* using the Best-model Containing W and Sz Indices

No.	*Compound*	*Exp. Activity*	*Estimated Activity*	*Residue*	*(Residue)^2*
1.	1	18.14	18.64	–0.50	0.25
2.	2	22.45	21.40	1.05	1.1025
3.	4	17.34	16.98	0.36	0.1296
4.	5	20.32	21.40	–1.08	1.1664
5.	6	22.78	22.60	0.18	0.0324

Σ(Residue)^2 = 2.6809

The predictive power of the models can be judged from quality factor Q. The Q-values are recorded in Table 4.1.5. The highest Q = 0.8139 for the model expressed by [eqn. (4.1.5)] indicates that it has highest predictive power. Further, conformation regarding predictive power is made by calculating predictive correlation coefficient, R^2_{pred}, which is obtained from the correlation between the observed and the estimated activity. The R^2_{pred} = 0.8906 confirms that the predictive power of the proposed model [eqn.(4.1.5)] is highest.

In support of our results we have also calculated three important statistical parameters: probable error of the coefficient of correlation (PE), least square error (LSE) and Friedman's lack of fit measure (LOF)[32–34]. These parameters are calculated from the following equations and summarized in Table 4.1.7.

$$PE = \frac{2}{3}\ \frac{1-r^2}{\sqrt{n}} \qquad (4.1.6)$$

where,

r – coefficient of correlation and n – number of compounds used.

$$LSE = \Sigma\,(Y_{obs} - Y_{calc-})^2 \qquad (4.1.7)$$

where,

Y_{obs} and Y_{calc} are the observed and calculated activities. In our case anti-bacterial activity of the sulfa drugs against *E. coli* –

$$LOF = \frac{LSE}{\{1-(C+d.p.)/n\}^2} \qquad (4.1.8)$$

where,

LSE – least square error, C – number of descriptors +1, p – number of independent parameters, n – number of compounds used, d – smoothing parameter which controls the bias in the scoring factor between equations with different number of terms and was kept 1.0.

Table 4.1.7: PE, LSE and LOF Values Calculated for the Derived Models for Modeling Antibacterial Activity of Sulfa Drugs against *E. coli*

Model	*TI*	*PE*	*LSE*	*LOF*
1.	W	0.1335	10.8149	67.5931
2.	Sz	0.0983	7.9653	49.7831
3.	$^1\chi$	0.1466	11.8836	74.2725
4.	J	0.2067	16.7492	104.6825
5.	logRB	0.1345	10.8994	68.1212
6.	W, J	0.1170	9.4800	14.8125
7.	Sz, J	0.0795	6.4424	10.0662
8.	$^1\chi$, J	0.1049	8.4976	13.2775
9.	J, logRB	0.1168	9.4683	14.7942
10.	W, Sz	0.0331	2.6809	4.1889
11.	W, $^1\chi$	0.1266	10.2637	16.0370
12.	Sz, $^1\chi$	0.0665	5.3842	8.4128

It is argued that if

r < PE, r is not significant;

r > PE, several times at least 3-times greater correlation is indicated

r > 6PE, correlation is definitely good.

The values of PE (Table 4.1.7) indicates that all the proposed correlations are definitely good and the one expressed by [eqn. (4.1.5)] is the best. The lowest value of both LSE and LOF are also in favour of the proposed model. It is important to mention that one should use LOF directly rather than LSE, the reason being LOF doesn't decrease with increased number of descriptors and the lowest value is found for an equation with the optimum number of parameters.

4.1.2.2. Anti-bacterial Activity of Sulfa Drugs against *K. penumonae*

As stated earlier only three sulfa drugs are effective against *K. pneumonae* and, therefore, it is not a good example for QSAR study. The data presented in Tables 4.1.4, 8, 9, 10 also indicate that this is not a good example for drug modeling. However, data did show that all the topological indices are equally worked and qualitatively the antibacterial activity[35] follow the sequence:

$$5 > 1 > 2 \qquad (4.1.9)$$

Table 4.1.8: Regression Analysis and Quality Correlation for Modeling Antibacterial Activity of Sulfa Drugs against *K. pneumonae*

No.	*TI (S)*	*Se*	*r(R)*	*F*	*Q*
1.	W	7.4458	0.3781	0.167	0.0508
2.	Sz	7.4458	0.3781	0.167	0.0508
3.	$^1\chi$	7.4458	0.3781	0.167	0.0508
4.	J	7.4458	–0.3781	0.167	–0.0508
5.	logBB	7.4458	0.3781	0.167	0.0508

Table 4.1.9: Found and Estimated Antibacterial Activity of Sulfa Drugs against *K. pneumonae* Using the Best Model Containing W Index

No.	*Compound*	*Exp. Activity*	*Estimated Activity*	*Residue*	*(Residue)²*
1.	1	27.85	27.85	0.00	0.00
2.	2	18.86	24.12	–5.26	27.6676
3.	5	29.39	24.12	5.27	27.7729

$\Sigma(\text{Residue})^2 = 55.4405$

4.1.2.3. Anti-bacterial Activity of Sulfa Drugs against *B. subtilis*

Like the case of *E. coli* here also five sulfa drugs are found active against *B. subtilis*. A perusal of Table 4.1.2 shows that the antibacterial activity of these five sulfa drugs follow the following sequence:

Table 4.1.10: PE, LSE and LOF Values Calculated for the Derived Models for Modeling Antibacterial Activity of Sulfa Drugs against *K. pneumonae*

Model	*TI*	*PE*	*LSE*	*LOF*
1.	W	0.3299	55.4405	124.5042
2.	Sz	0.3299	55.4405	124.5042
3.	$^1\chi$	0.3299	55.4405	124.5042
4.	J	0.3299	55.4405	124.5042
5.	logRB	0.3299	55.4405	124.5042

$$2 > 1 > 4 > 5 > 3 \tag{4.1.10}$$

However, this sequence doesn't establish any structure-activity relationship. Consequently, we have undertaken simple and multiple linear regression analysis. The correlation matrix (Table 4.1.4) indicates that here Balaban index (J) is capable of giving statistically significant mono-para-metric model. The regression parameters of J is the only topological index capable of yielding statistically significant mono-parametric model. This model is found as below:

Anti-bacterial activity against *B. sibtilis* = 44.9398 - 12.0593 (± 6.0957) J (4.1.11)

$n = 5$, $Se = 3.3139$, $r = -0.7524$, $F = 3.9140$, $Q = 0.2270$

This shows that anti-bacterial activities of sulfa drugs against *B. subtilis* are inversely proportional to the magnitude of J index. This J index is the extended connectivity index, indicating there by that extended connectivity is not favourable for the exhibition of the activity against the bacteria used.

Table 4.1.11: Regression Analysis and Quality of Correlation for Modeling Antibacterial Activity of Sulfa Drugs against *B. subtilis*

Model	*TI*	*Se*	R^2_A	*R*	*F*	*Q*
1	W	4.5904	–	0.4092	0.603	0.0891
2.	Sz	4.6432	–	0.3849	0.522	0.0829
3.	$^1\chi$	4.2990	–	0.5194	1.1080	0.1208
4.	J	3.3139	–	–0.7524	3.914	0.2270
5.	logRB	4.5885	–	0.4100	0.606	0.0893
6.	W, J	3.5663	0.3300	0.8155	1.985	0.2287
7.	Sz, J	3.7330	0.2659	0.7956	1.724	0.2131
8.	$^1\chi$, J	3.6322	0.3050	0.8078	1.878	0.2224
9.	J, logRB	3.5681	0.3293	0.8153	1.982	0.2285
10.	W, Sz	5.5789	–0.6397	0.4245	0.220	0.0761
11.	W, $^1\chi$	3.3067	0.4240	0.8438	2.472	0.2552
12.	Sz, $^1\chi$	4.3323	0.0112	0.7111	1.023	0.1641

Once again following the "Rule of Thumb" we have ultimately made bi-parametric regression analysis. The results recorded in Table 4.1.11 show that all the attempted bi-parametric regressions resulted into statistically significant models and that the model containing W and $^1\chi$ is the best model. This model is found as below:

Anti-bacterial activity against *B.subtilis* = 94.2415 + 23.1249 (± 11.8920) $^1\chi$ - 0.1250 (± 0.0719) W (4.1.12)

n = 5, Se = 3.3067, r = 0.8438, R^2_A = 0.4240, F = 2.472, Q = 0.2552

The positive coefficient of first-order connectivity ($^1\chi$) indicates that first-order branching is favourable for the exhibition of the activity. The Wiener index (W) accounts for the shape and size, the negative coefficient of which indicates their unfavourable contribution in the exhibition of the activity.

Table 4.1.12: Found and Estimated Antibacterial Activity of Sulfa Drug against *B. subtilis* using the Best-Model Containing W and $^1\chi$ Indices

No.	Compound	Exp. Activity	Estimated Activity	Residue	$(Residue)^2$
1.	1	25.10	25.00	0.10	0.01
2.	2	25.90	22.67	3.23	10.4329
3.	3	15.45	15.43	0.02	0.0004
4.	4	19.80	19.77	0.03	0.0009
5.	5	19.29	22.67	–3.38	11.4244

$\Sigma(\text{Residue})^2$ =21.8686

Table 4.1.13: PE, LSE and LOF Values Calculated for the Derived Models for Modeling Antibacterial Activity of Sulfa Drugs against *B. subtilis*

Model	TI	PE	LSE	LOF
1.	W	0.2482	63.2164	395.1025
2.	Sz	0.2540	64.6773	404.2331
3.	$^1\chi$	0.2177	55.4429	346.5181
4.	J	0.1294	32.9464	205.9150
5.	logRB	0.2480	63.1637	394.7731
6.	W, J	0.0998	25.4372	39.7456
7.	Sz, J	0.1094	27.8700	43.5468
8.	$^1\chi$, J	0.1036	26.3851	41.2267
9.	J, logRB	0.0999	25.4627	39.7854
10.	W, Sz	0.2444	62.2481	97.2626
11.	W, $^1\chi$	0.0858	21.8686	34.1696
12.	Sz, $^1\chi$	0.1474	37.5382	58.6534

As in the case of *E. coli,* here also we have used Q and R^2_{pred} to estimate predictive power of the model. Table 4.1.11 shows that Q value is the highest for the model expressed by [eqn. (4.1.12)]. Also, the value of 0.8280 for R^2_{pred} supports this finding. Furthermore, the comparison of found and calculated activity (Table 4.1.12), and the lowest values of LSE and LOF (Table 4.1.13) are in favour of the proposed model [eqn. (4.1.12)].

4.1.3. Conclusions

From the results and discussion made above we conclude that the distance-based topological indices can be used successfully for modeling anti-bacterial activity of sulfa drugs against *E. coli* and *B. subtilis*. However, the set of topological indices used are not good for modeling the activity against *K. pneumonae*. The results also show that different topological indices are responsible for giving statistical significant QSAR models for different bacteria used.

4.2. Synthesis and QSAR Study on Antibacterial Activity of Mannich Bases: Molecular vs Rooted Graphs

4.2.1. Introduction

Of late it has been known that Mannich reaction not only provides an important biosynthetic route for natural product but also to several organic compounds acting as drugs[1]. Notable application of Mannich bases is in the field of pharmaceutical and medicinal chemistry. As many as 40 per cent publications on Mannich bases are concern with these fields and is evident from the Tetrahedron report[2]. Both these publications[1,2] provide elaborate treatment of the recent synthetic trends together with applicability of Mannich bases as antineoplastic drugs, analgesics, antibiotics, CNS stimulant, antiarrythmic, antiinflammatory, antimalarials, antifungal, insecticidal, pesticidal, germicidal, herbicidal, fungicidal, antihypertensive, antitumor, anticonvulsant, antileufemotic, anticoagulant, hypoglycemic, antiprotozal etc. agents. In addition, Mannich bases exhibit technological applications also. Some such applications being in polymer chemistry, paints surface active agents, corrosion inhibitors, fuel additives, levelling agents, dispersants, stabilizers and ashless detergent additives for fuels, coagulants, polishing of brass etc.[1,2].

Prompted by the aforementioned versatile applications of Mannich bases we have earlier synthesized Mannich bases[3–16] of flubendazole, mebendazole, albendazole and some sulfa drugs and screen them for their antimicrobiol activity, particularly antibacterial activity. In continuation of our earlier work on Mannich bases the present communication deals with synthesis, characterization, and Quantitative Structure-Activity Relationship (QSAR) studies on Mannich bases derived from Nicotinoyl-4-aminobenzamido-methyl-amines (Figure 4.2.1) using a series of distance-based topological indices: Wiener (W)-[17] first-order olecular connectivity ($^1\chi$)-[18], Balaban (J)-[19], Szeged (Sz)-[20,21] and logRB-indices. The details of these indices can be further traced in the excellent reviews and books[22–27]. The QSAR models were obtained by regression analysis following the maximum R^2-method[28]. While the predictive power of the proposed models were examined by the quality factor Q[29–34].

Figure 4.2.1: General Structures for the Newly Synthesis Mannich Bases.

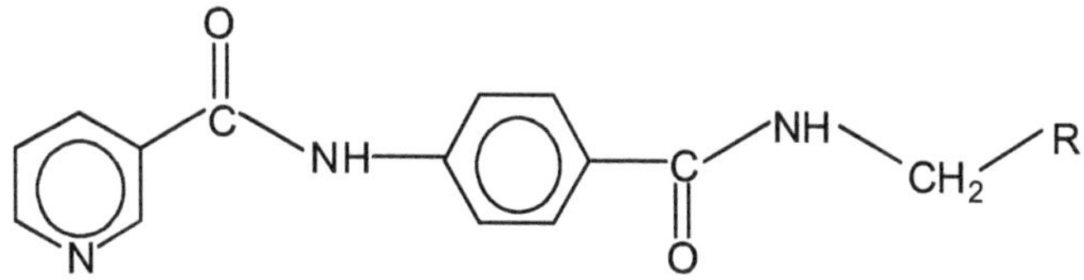

(1) R =

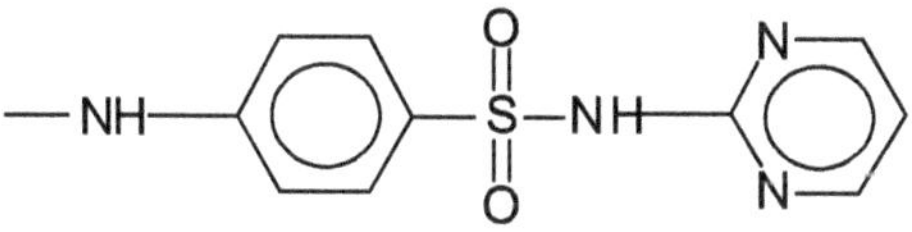

(2) R =

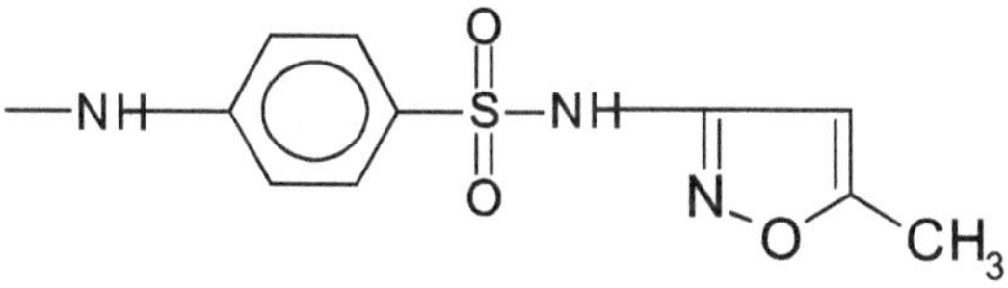

(3) R =

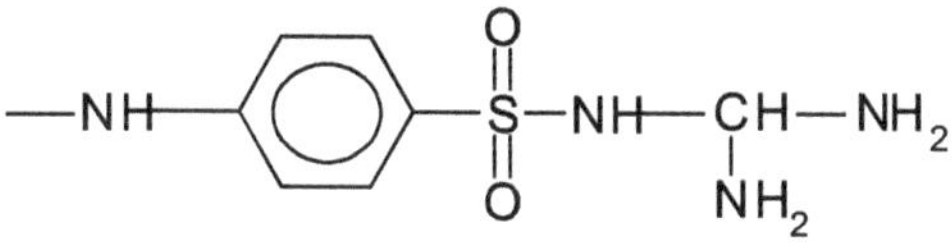

(4) R =

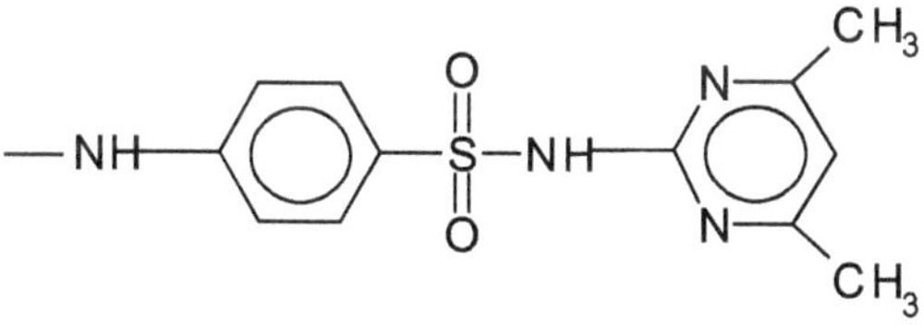

(5) R =

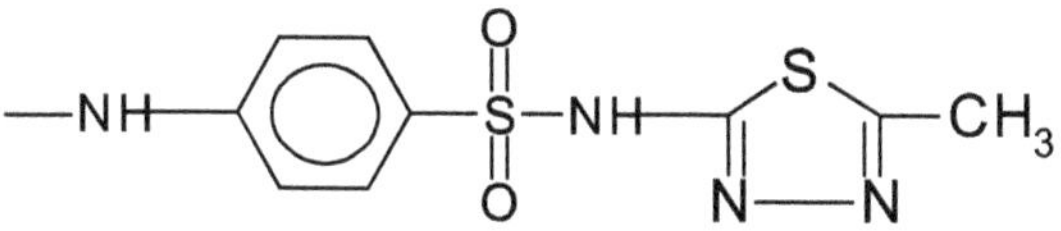

(6) R =

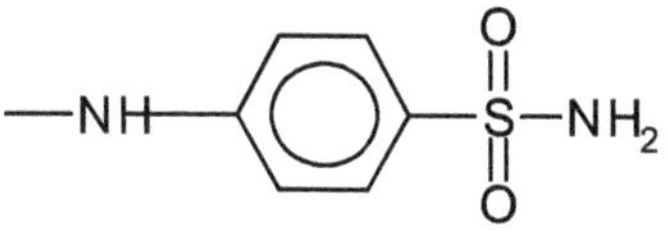

Contd...

Figure 4.2.1–*Contd...*

(7) $R = -N(CH_3)_2$

(8) $R = -N(CH_2-CH_3)_2$

(9) $R = -N(C_6H_5)_2$

(10) $R = -N(CH_2-CH_2OH)_2$

(11) $R = -N(C_4H_8O)$ (morpholino)

(12) $R = -N(C_4H_8)N-CH_2-NH-C(=O)-C_6H_4-NH-C(=O)-C_5H_4N$

4.2.2. Results and Discussion

All the twelve Mannich bases were synthesised employing the method reported earlier and were characterized by elemental analysis, TLC, uv, ir and nmr studies.

4.2.2.1. UV Spectral Study

The details for recording uv spectra of the Mannich bases is given in the experimental section. All the Mannich bases exhibited a band at 210 ± 5 nm due to the presence of amido moiety.

In addition, bands at 219 ± 5 nm and 257 ± 2 nm were indicative of the presence of sulphoxide, benzene chromophore and pyridine nucleus respectively. Moreover, the band at 260 ± 2 nm was attributed to be due to the presence of sulfonamide moiety.

4.2.2.2. Ir Spectral Study

Due to the huge molecular structure of the synthesised Mannich bases complete ir spectra data are not discussed. Furthermore, our objective is not to make detail vibrational analysis as well as we are not interested at present to undergo normal coordinate analysis. Our primary objective was to characterize the newly synthesised Mannich bases. Consequently, we have summarized important i.r. bands (Table 4.2.1) and discussed important among them, thus characterizing the Mannich bases. The results can be summarised as below.

Table 4.2.1: Ir Frequency Bands of Nicotinoyl-4-amino Benzamidomethyl Amines

	II	III	IV	V	VI	VII	VIII	IX	X	XI	XII
	3500(w)	3450(w)	3500(w)	3440(w)	3420(w)	3400(m)	3430(m)	3420(s)	3400(s)	3450(s)	3300(w)
[illegible]	3380(m)	3350(s)	3350(s)	3340(w)	3150(m)	3200(w)	3200(w)	3300(w)	2950(w)	3300(w)	3199(w)
[illegible]280(m)	3150(m)	3200(s)	3200(m)	3180(m)	3050(m)	3010(w)	3000(s)	3010(w)	2880	3050(w)	2910(w)
3110(m)	2950(w)	3050(m)	3050(w)	3050(m)	2920(w)	2950(w)	2850(m)	2915(s)	2780(w)	2940(w)	2800(w)
3060(s)	2830(w)	2950(w)	2960(w)	2930(w)	2800(w)	2915(w)	2750(w)	2850(m)	1665(m)	2870(w)	2750(w)
2950(s)	1665(s)	2800(w)	2955(w)	1660(m)	1660(m)	2840(w)	1665(m)	2805(w)	1600(m)	2790(w)	1657(m)
2885(s)	1620(s)	1670(m)	2790(w)	1600(s)	1600(s)	2775(w)	1600(m)	2780(w)	1515(w)	1665(m)	1620(sh)
2810(s)	1599(s)	1620(m)	1655(m)	1520(s)	1520(s)	1660(s)	1530(m)	1660(s)	1450(w)	1601(s)	1598(s)
2750(m)	1510(s)	1600(m)	1630(m)	1410(s)	1450(s)	1600(s)	1465(w)	1620(w)	1415	1565(m)	1520(s)
1655(s)	1465(s)	1530(s)	1600(m)	1390(m)	1410(s)	1525(s)	1458(w)	1600(s)	1320(w)	1530(m)	1473(w)
1600(s)	1409(s)	1410(s)	1550(m)	1325(w)	1315(m)	1460(m)	1415(m)	1525(s)	1245(w)	1455(s)	1467(w)
1585(s)	1389(s)	1380(w)	1505(m)	1280(s)	1265(w)	1410(s)	1390(m)	1450(s)	1190	1425(m)	1429(m)
1550(m)	1320(s)	1310(m)	1440(m)	1190(w)	1250(w)	1320(m)	1320(m)	1415(s)	1125(w)	1309(s)	1319(m)
1448(s)	1269(s)	1235(m)	1410(m)	1140(m)	1190(w)	1268(m)	1260(m)	1310(s)	1099(m)	1230(w)	1250(m)
1495(s)	1190(s)	1235(m)	1385(s)	1115(w)	1149(s)	1182	1190	1225(w)	1065(s)	1191	1180
1415(s)	1160(s)	1175(s)	1349(s)	1090(w)	1090(m)	1150(m)	1112(w)	1180	1030(w)	1109	1110(m)
1329(s)	1149(sh)	1130(s)	1310(s)	1045(w)	1040(m)	1110(m)	1045(w)	1100(s)	940(m)	1050(s)	1087(m)
1265(s)	1095(s)	1089(s)	1265(m)	1030(w)	1020(w)	1090(w)	1020(w)	1045(s)	900(w)	900(s)	1040(m)
1220(m)	1030(s)	1055(m)	1190(s)	1000(w)	990(w)	1050(s)	900(m)	895(s)	850(w)	875(s)	1025(m)
1190(m)	1005(s)	1030(w)	1150(s)	900(m)	958(w)	1040(s)	850(m)	870(s)	828(s)	828(w)	982(w)
1158(s)	925(s)	900(m)	1080(w)	850(w)	900(m)	1025(s)	800(w)	800(m)	802(m)	770(w)	950(m)
1130(m)	898(m)	825(s)	1030(w)	830(w)	825(m)	995(w)	765(s)	762(m)	760(w)	690(m)	865(m)

Contd...

Table 4.2.1–Contd...

I	II	III	IV	V	VI	VII	VIII	IX	X	XI	XII
1100(s)	829(s)	790(w)	1000(w)	809(m)	802(m)	958(w)	700(m)	690(m)	700(w)		845(w)
1010(m)	765(w)	770(w)	978(s)	765(s)	765(s)	925(w)	670(s)		655(m)		825(w)
975(w)	735(w)	730(w)	900(m)	695(s)	698(m)	898(s)					810(w)
940(s)	680(s)	688(s)	855(m)		670(m)	850(s)					760(m)
840(m)			830(m)			820(s)					745(m)
820(w)			785(s)			765(s)					690(s)
795(s)			770(sh)			750(sh)					
715(m)			700(s)			695(s)					
680(s)			670(s)								

(m) = medium, (s) = strong, (w) = weak, (sh) = shoulder.

Medium to strong characteristic N-H band due to secondary amide group appeared at 3450 ± 50 cm^{-1}. A medium band at 3350 ± 50 cm^{-1} may be attributed to the presence of sulfonamide moiety. The bands due to C-H stretching, deformation and bending are observed at 2940 ± 20 cm^{-1} (asymmetric –C-H), 2840 ± 40 cm^{-1} (symmetric C-H), 1540 ± 15 cm^{-1} and 2820 ± 50 cm^{-1} respectively. The aromatic =C-H, C-C and C-N ring stretching vibrations occurred at 3050 ± 50 cm^{-1}, 1495 ± 10 cm^{-1}, 1420 ± 20 cm^{-1} respectively. The inplane bending vibrations due to heteroatomic ring were exhibited at 1180 ± 10 cm^{-1} and 1100 – 1020 cm^{-1}. On the other hand out-of-plane =C-H bending vibrations appear at 850 ± 30 cm^{-1} and 680 ± 10 cm^{-1}, due to 3-substituted pyridine. The presence of CH_2N< group is indicated by a band at 2780 ± 30 cm^{-1}. A strong to medium intensity vibration of carbonyl stretches is indicated by a band at 1660 ± 10 cm^{-1}, and is due to secondary amide group. The N-H bending vibrations are assigned at 1600 ± 20 cm^{-1}. This also is due to secondary amide group. The bands at 1310 ± 10 cm^{-1}, 750 ± 20 cm^{-1} are due to N-H bending and wagging respectively. The symmetrical stretching of S=O group is indicated by a band at 1175 ± 10 cm^{-1}.

Table 4.2.2: ^{1}H NMR Spectral Data of Nicotinoyl-4-minobenzamidomethyl Amines

Compd. No.	*δ values in ppm*					
	CH_2 (d)	*NH (s)*	*Various (m) Ring Protons*	*CONH of Ring I (s)*	*CONH of Ring II (t)*	*SO_2NH (s)*
1	2.71	6.15	6.5 – 7.9	7.71	8.25	10.9
2	2.82	6.10	6.8 – 7.8	7.40	8.30	11.0
3	2.50	6.15	6.55 – 7.9	7.70	8.25	10.8
4	2.50	6.10	6.5 – 7.6	7.80	8.40	10.8
5	2.75	6.10	6.5 – 7.8	7.40	8.30	10.8
6	2.75	5.85	6.6 – 7.8	7.70	8.30	10.9
7	2.75	–	7.1 – 7.85	7.71	8.25	–
8	2.51	–	7.2 – 7.8	7.70	8.30	–
9	2.50	–	6.9 – 7.8	7.70	8.20	–
10	2.65	–	6.9 – 7.9	7.70	8.30	–
11	2.70	–	7.3 – 7.8	7.70	8.30	–
12	2.50	–	7.2 – 7.8	7.70	8.30	–

(d) = doublet; (s) = singlet; (m) = multiplet; (t) = triplet.

In addition to the above, vibrations due to C-H in-plane bending, due to 1,4-disubstituted benzene is indicated by a bands at 1250 ± 15 cm^{-1}, 1150 ± 40 cm^{-1} and 1010 ± 10 cm^{-1}. Here, out-of-plane bending due to 3-substituted pyridine are overlapped. The aromatic six-membered ring vibrations are exhibited at 950 ± 50 cm^{-1}.

The above ir spectral data, therefore, characterize the structure of newly synthesised Mannich bases (Figure 4.2.1).

4.2.2.3. Nmr Spectral Study

Further characterization of the Mannich bases is carried out by ^1H nmr data (Table 4.2.2). The details of nmr recording is given in the experimental section. All the Mannich bases show magnetic resonance due to N-H protons, alkyl protons, aryl ring protons as well as heteroaryl protons. The characteristic resonance due to CH_2 protons were exhibits in the region δ 5.85 – 6.1 ppm (J = 8.57 Hz) as a doublet. The sharp singlet due to NH of sulfonamide moiety is observed in the region δ 5.85 – 6.1 ppm. The singlet at δ 6.8 ppm (J = 9.64 Hz) as doublet is observed due to H ortho to NH. Another peak due to H at 5th position in pyridine ring is observed as a double at δ 7.35 ppm. In the region δ 7.55 – 7.6 ppm (J = 9.64 Hz) a doublet due to H ortho to sulfonamide moiety (SO_2) is observed. A singlet peak is seen in the region δ 7.7 – 7.73 ppm due to CONH of ring – I is observed. Proton resonance due to H ortho to >C=O is observed at δ 7.79 ppm (J = 11.42 Hz) as doublet. In the region δ 8.1 – 8.2 ppm a complex series of lines are obtained which are attributed H para to heteroatom in pyridine ring. The triplet for CONH of ring-II is exhibited in the region δ 8.25 – 8.3 ppm (J = 9.64 Hz). A doublet at δ 8.38 – 8.77 ppm is due to proton at 6-position in pyridine ring. Similarly, a strong doublet is observed at δ 9.2 ppm due to proton at 2nd position in the pyridine ring, while a sharp singlet is observed in the region δ 10.9 – 11.0 ppm for SO_2NH of sulfonamide moiety. In addition, other nmr peaks due to ring structure are also observed. These peaks vary due to changes in the structure of the Mannich bases.

4.2.2.4. Antimicrobial Study

All the twelve Mannich bases were screened for their antibacterial potential and the exhibited significant response against *E. coli*, *K. pneumonae* and *B. subtilis*. No inhibitory effect was shown by them against *P. aeruginusa*, *S. typhosa* and *S. aureus*. The details of antimicrobiol screening is described in details under experimental section. However, the results obtained are presented in Table 4.2.3. A close look at Table 4.2.3, gives the following order of antibacterial activities of the Mannich bases against the three bacteria.

E. coli

$$5 > 1 > 4 > 6 > 7 > 11 > 8 > 2 > 9 > 10 > 12 > 13 \quad \textbf{(4.2.1)}$$

K. pneumonae

$$10 > 1 > 8 > 7 > 6 > 2 > 12 > 11 \quad \textbf{(4.2.2)}$$

B. subtilis

$$1 > 2 > 4 \quad \textbf{(4.2.3)}$$

However, the above sequences doesn't give any structure-activity relationships. In view of this we have undertaken topological modeling of antibacterial activities of Mannich bases against these three bacteria. The results are discussed in the following section.

4.2.2.5. Structure-Activity Relationship (SAR)

At this stage it is worth to mention that topological indices are graph invariants obtained from the molecular graphs[22–27]. These indices are considered as numerical

Table 4.2.3: Antibacterial Activity of Mannich Bases under Present Study

Compound No.	Zone of Inhibition in mm				Average
	Concentration in μg/ml				
	10	20	40	80	
(A) Against *E. coli*					
1	10.46	10.66	13.70	18.70	13.38
2	11.33	11.56	11.83	13.46	12.05
3	10.96	11.43	11.06	11.70	11.29
4	11.43	13.90	13.70	14.10	13.28
5	12.43	14.93	14.,43	15.06	14.21
6	13.13	12.76	13.20	13.20	13.07
7	13.30	10.86	12.63	14.56	12.84
8	13.46	12.20	11.90	11.56	12.28
9	11.53	11.90	12.43	11.06	11.73
10	9.00	11.76	12.40	13.66	11.70
11	11.96	11.66	13.13	14.56	12.83
12	12.16	11.80	11.03	10.26	11.31
(B) Against *K. pneumonae*					
1	18.93	18.30	19.23	20.96	19.35
2	12.56	14.73	14.43	13.70	13.85
6	11.10	12.00	13.76	21.40	14.56
7	10.90	12.06	17.26	18.56	14.70
8	12.83	14.76	15.10	17.63	15.08
10	28.00	25.20	22.06	27.46	25.68
11	12.23	11.13	13.60	16.30	13.44
12	12.43	14.43	14.80	13.70	13.84
(C) Against *B. subtilis*					
1	15.43	20.40	22.93	25.36	21.03
2	14.10	18.63	20.70	23.50	19.23
4	6.00	11.26	13.66	17.63	12.14

representation of molecular structure. Thus, 1: 1 correlation between structure and activity is possible using topological indices. The molecular graphs used for their calculations are obtained by deleting all the carbon-hydrogen as well as heteroatom-hydrogen bonds from the molecular structure. Thus, imposing certain conditions on the molecular graphs, a particular topological index is derived. In our case we have used a series of distance-based topological indices: Wiener (W)-[17], Szeged (Sz)-[20,21], first-order molecular connectivity ($^1\chi$)-[18], Balaban (J)-[19] and logRB indices[22–27]. These indices have been calculated for the complete graph of the Mannich bases as well as for rooted graphs. Since, the Mannich bases are obtained due to variation in R, they are rooted at R; thus separating R. The R skeleton, therefore, represents the rooted graph of the Mannich bases. In view of this our Quantitative Structure-Activity Relationship (QSAR) study is carried out in two different ways: (i) QSAR considering the entire graph representation of Mannich bases and (ii) QSAR considering rooted graph *i.e.*, R-skeleton of the Mannich bases. Such a study will help us knowing the role of R-skeleton of the Mannich bases on their antibacterial activity[35]. The results are, therefore, discussed separately under these two headings. The topological indices calculated for them are given in Table 4.2.4 and 4.2.5.

Table 4.2.4: Distance Based Topological Indices Calculated for Mannich Bases Ysed in the Present Study

Compound No.	*W*	*Sz*	$^1\chi$	*J*	*logRB*
1	5390	7745	17.4038	1.0673	1178.2830
2	5389	7544	17.2977	1.0683	1177.8770
3	4212	5928	15.7400	1.2697	953.5831
4	6234	8957	18.1915	1.0780	1338.9600
5	5389	7544	17.2977	1.0683	1177.8770
6	3203	4577	14.3255	1.2680	753.0981
7	1259	1790	10.5585	1.6548	338.8745
8	1629	2250	11.6346	1.6464	425.2686
9	3441	4944	15.7035	1.2005	844.4610
10	2057	2768	12.6346	1.6458	522.6647
11	1832	2696	12.2203	1.3151	470.0750
12	10002	14496	21.4407	0.8875	1951.7250

Table 4.2.5: Distance Based Topological Indices Calculated from Rooted Graphs of Mannich Bases Used in the Present Ctudy

Compound No.	*W*	*Sz*	$^1\chi$	*J*	*logRB*
1	536	818	8.0773	1.8372	162.0572
2	535	731	7.9712	1.8479	161.6517
3	307	427	6.4155	2.4613	96.2437
4	722	1092	8.8650	1.8868	215.2262
5	535	731	7.9712	1.8479	161.6517
6	152	236	4.9990	2.3936	48.2757
7	4	4	1.4142	1.6330	0.6931
8	20	20	2.4142	2.1906	5.6630
9	264	444	6.4495	1.6872	81.3185
10	56	56	3.4142	2.4478	17.0297
11	27	54	3.0000	2.0000	7.4547
12	1832	2696	12.0223	1.3151	470.0750

4.2.3. QSAR Study Considering Entire Molecular Graph of Mannich Bases

For making QSAR study considering the entire molecular graphs of Mannich bases we will use their antibacterial activities presented in Table 4.2.3 and the topological indices presented in Table 4.2.4. It is worthy to mention that the topological indices used here belong to first (W, Sz) and second ($^1\chi$, J, logRB) generation topological indices. Therefore, degeneracy (more than one values) is observed in their cases.

Table 4.2.6: Correlation Matrix for Modeling Antibacterial Activity of Mannich Bases Considering Entire Molecular Graphs

	Activity	*W*	*Sz*	*$^1\chi$*	*J*	*logRB*
(A) For *E. coli*						
Activity	1.0000					
W	–0.0901	1.0000				
Sz	–0.0915	0.9996	1.0000			
$^1\chi$	–0.0550	0.9749	0.9724	1.0000		
J	–0.1193	–0.8780	–0.8784	–0.9310	1.0000	
LogRB	–0.0732	0.9973	0.9961	0.9882	–0.8991	1.0000
(B) For *K. pneumonae*						
Activity	1.0000					
W	–0.1966	1.0000				
Sz	–0.2068	0.9997	1.0000			
$^1\chi$	–0.1455	0.9840	0.9817	1.0000		
J	0.3508	–0.8835	–0.8850	–0.9247	1.0000	
logRB	–0.1836	0.9984	0.9974	0.9923	–0.8990	1.0000
(C) For *B. subtilis*						
Activity	1.0000					
W	–0.98130	1.0000				
Sz	–0.94780	0.99145	1.0000			
$^1\chi$	–0.96858	0.99834	0.99732	1.0000		
J	–0.99418	0.99633	0.97664	0.98974	1.0000	
logRB	–0.98107	1.00000	0.99160	0.99841	0.99623	1.0000

Since the different number of Mannich bases are active against the three bacteria used we have obtained separate correlation matrices for them. These matrices give intercorrelatedness between the topological indices and their corrections with the antibacterial activities. Such matrices are presented in Table 4.2.6, which shows that the topological indices are highly linearly correlated. It means that QSAR model containing any combination of these indices will suffer due to collinearity defect. However, such a problem can be resolved easily using Randic recommendations. The correlation matrices also show that none of the topological indices correlates singly with the antibacterial activity against *E. coli* and *K. pneumonae*. However, the results did show that the Balaban index (J) is a better topological index for modeling antibacterial activity of the Mannich bases against these two bacteria. In case of *B. subtilis* all the topological indices are excellently correlated with the activity. This perhaps may be due to a very small number (three) of Mannich bases active against this bacteria.

4.2.3.1. Antibacterial activity against *E. coli*

The quality of correlation and regression parameters (Table 4.2.7) for antibacterial activity against *E. coli* show that none of the topological indices when used singly are capable of giving any statistical significant model. However, the results did show that statistics is improved when we carried out bi-parametric regression analysis. The best bi-parametric model for modeling antibacterial activity against *E. coli* was the one contains $^1\chi$ and J as the correlating parameters. This model is found as:

$$\text{Antibacterial activity against } E.\ coli = 23.6971 - 0.3575\ (\pm 0.2310)\ ^1\chi - 4.5117\ (\pm 2.8392)\ J \quad (4.2.4)$$

$n = 12$, $Se = 0.8930$, $r = 0.4705$, $R^2_A = 0.0484$, $F = 1.2799$, $Q = 0.5269$

We have, therefore, carried out a detailed statistical analysis and the results are presented in Tables 4.2.7 to 4.2.9. All these results show that the model is not a very good model for *E. coli*.

Table 4.2.7: Regression Analysis and Quality of Correlations for Modeling Antibacterial Activity of Mannich Bases against *E. coli* Considering Entire Molecular Graphs

Model	*Topological Index*	*Se*	R^2_A	*R*	*F*	*Q*
1	W	0.9563	–	–0.0901	0.0818	0.0942
2	Sz	0.9562	–	–0.0915	0.0845	0.0957
3	$^1\chi$	0.9587	–	–0.0550	0.0303	0.0573
4	J	0.9533	–	–0.1193	0.1444	0.1251
5	logRB	0.9576	–	–0.0732	0.0538	0.0764
6	W, J	0.9166	–0.0023	0.4241	0.9871	0.4626
7	Sz, J	0.9148	0.0014	0.4278	1.0079	0.4676
8	$^1\chi$, J	0.8930	0.0484	0.4705	1.2799	0.5269
9	J, logRB	0.9142	0.0029	0.4291	1.0159	0.4693
10	W, Sz	1.0066	–0.2088	0.1045	0.0497	0.1038
11	W, $^1\chi$	0.9969	–0.1857	0.1728	0.1385	0.1733
12	Sz, $^1\chi$	0.9970	–0.1860	0.1721	0.1373	0.1726

Regression parameters under sub-classes -

Class I: Containing Mannich bases 2,3,9,11,12

$n = 5$, $Se = 0.08731$, $R^2_A = 0.9812$, $R = 0.9975$, $F = 105.1819$, $Q = 11.4261$

Class II: Containing Mannich bases 1,4,5,6,7,8,10

$n = 7$, $Se = 0.4084$, $R^2_A = 0.7445$, $R = 0.9109$, $F = 9.7435$, $Q = 2.2304$

Table 4.2.8: Found and Estimated Antibacterial Activity of Mannich Bases against *E. coli* Using Best Model Containing $^1\chi$, J as well as Considering Entire Molecular Graphs

Compound No.	*Found*	*Estimated*	*Residue*	*(Residue)^2*
1	13.38	12.62	0.76	0.5776
2	12.05	12.69	–0.64	0.4096
3	11.29	12.34	–1.05	1.1025
4	13.28	12.33	0.95	0.9025
5	14.21	12.69	1.52	2.3104
6	13.07	12.85	0.22	0.0484
7	12.84	12.45	0.39	0.1521
8	12.28	12.11	0.17	0.0289
9	11.73	12.66	–0.93	0.8649
10	11.70	11.75	–0.05	0.0025
11	12.83	13.39	–0.56	0.3136
12	11.31	12.07	–0.76	0.5776

$\Sigma(\text{Residue})^2 = 7.1785$

Table 4.2.9: PE, LSE, LOF Values Calculated for the Derived Models for Modeling Antibacterial Activity of Mannich Bases against *E. coli* as well as Considering Entire Graph

Model	*Topological Index*	*PE*	*LSE*	*LOF*
1	W	0.1908	9.1454	329.23
2	Sz	0.1908	9.1429	329.14
3	$^1\chi$	0.1918	9.1923	330.92
4	J	0.1896	9.0889	327.20
5	logRB	0.1914	9.1708	330.14
6	W, J	0.1578	7.5615	68.05
7	Sz, J	0.1572	7.5329	67.79
8	$^1\chi$, J	0.1498	7.1785	64.60
9	J, logRB	0.1570	7.5219	67.69
10	W, Sz	0.1903	9.1194	82.07
11	W, $^1\chi$	0.1866	8.9447	88.50
12	Sz, $^1\chi$	0.1867	8.9471	80.52

In order to understand better relationship between structure and activity we have correlated each of the topological index and the activity against *E. coli* and observed that the data set could be divided into two sub-classes I and II containing Mannich bases 2, 3, 9, 11, 12 under sub class I and 1, 4, 5, 6, 7, 8, 10 under sub-class II. When we carried out regression analysis under these sub-classes we observed that excellent statistics in both the classes is obtained under bi-parametric regression contains ${}^1\chi$ and J as the correlating parameters. The details are given below:

Sub-class I

$$\text{Activity against } E.\ coli = 20.2129 - 0.5434\ (\pm 0.0429)\ {}^1\chi - 8.1997\ (\pm 0.8285)\ J \qquad (4.2.5)$$

n = 5, Se = 0.0873, r = 0.9975, R^2_A = 0.9812, F = 105.1819, Q = 11.4261

Sub-class II

$$\text{Activity against } E.\ coli = 25.9294 - 0.3481\ (\pm 0.2015)\ {}^1\chi - 5.8511\ (\pm 2.1247)\ J \qquad (4.2.6)$$

n = 7, Se = 0.4084, r = 0.9109, R^2_A = 0.7445, F = 9.7435, Q = 2.2304

4.2.3.2. Antibacterial Activity against *K. pneumonae*

We now discuss antibacterial activity against *K. pneumonae*. As stated earlier only eight Mannich bases are active against this bacteria and that the sequence expressed by eqn. (4.2.2) doesn't establish any structure-activity relationship. Consequently, we have again used topological indices for modeling antibacterial activity of Mannich bases against this bacteria. The results as recorded in Tables 4.2.10 to 4.2.12 indicates again that no monoparametric models are possible and that

Table 4.2.10: Regression Analysis and Quality of Correlations for Modeling Antibacterial Activity of Mannich Bases against *K. pneumonae* Considering Entire Graph

Model	Topological Index	Se	R^2_A	R	F	Q
1	W	4.4680	–	–0.19662	0.2413	0.0440
2	Sz	4.4584	–	–0.2068	0.2682	0.0464
3	${}^1\chi$	4.5084	–	–0.1455	0.1297	0.0322
4	J	4.2674	–	0.3508	0.8418	0.0822
5	logRB	4.4795	–	–0.1836	0.2093	0.0410
6	W, J	4.5161	–0.1458	0.4260	0.5548	0.0943
7	Sz, J	4.5408	–0.1584	0.4154	0.5214	0.0915
8	${}^1\chi$, J	4.0435	0.0814	0.5864	1.3101	0.1450
9	J, logRB	4.4269	–0.1010	0.4621	0.6788	0.1044
10	W, Sz	4.4073	–0.0913	0.4695	0.7071	0.1065
11	W, ${}^1\chi$	4.7054	–0.2439	0.3339	0.3137	0.0071
12	Sz, ${}^1\chi$	4.6449	–0.2121	0.3663	0.3874	0.0834

Regression parameters under sub-classes -

Class I: Containing Mannich bases 2,7,8,12

n = 4, Se = 0.1608, R^2_A = 0.9333, R = 0.9888, F = 22.0020, Q = 5.8041

Class II: Containing Mannich bases 1,6,10,11

n = 4, Se = 2.6162, R^2_A = 0.7796, R = 0.9626, F = 6.3060, Q = 0.3679

bi-parametric model contains $^1\chi$ and J gives better statistics. This model is found as below:

$$\text{Antibacterial activity against } K.\ pneumonae = -31.7149 + 1.4021 (\pm 1.0807)\ ^1\chi + 20.7946 (\pm 12.2601)\ J \qquad (4.2.7)$$

$n = 8$, $Se = 4.0435$, $r = 0.5864$, $R^2_A = 0.0814$, $F = 1.3101$, $Q = 0.1450$

Table 4.2.11: Found and Estimated Antibacterial Activity of Mannich Bases against *K. pneumonae* Using Best Model Containing $^1\chi$, J as well as Considering Entire Molecular Graph

Compound No.	*Found*	*Estimated*	*Residue*	*(Residue)^2*
1	19.35	15.17	4.18	17.4724
2	13.85	14.74	–0.89	0.7921
6	14.56	14.73	–0.17	0.0289
7	14.70	17.49	–2.79	7.7841
8	15.08	18.82	–3.74	13.9875
10	25.68	20.22	5.46	29.8116
11	13.44	12.76	0.68	0.4624
12	13.84	16.79	–2.95	8.7025

$\Sigma(\text{Residue})^2 = 81.7526$

Table 4.2.12: PE, LSE, LOF Values Calculated for the Derived Models for Modeling Antibacterial Activity of Mannich Bases against *K. pneumonae* as well as Considering Entire Molecular Graph

Model	*Topological Index*	*PE*	*LSE*	*LOF*
1	W	0.2250	119.7785	1916.45
2	Sz	0.2240	119.2652	1908.24
3	$^1\chi$	0.2291	121.9576	1951.32
4	J	0.2052	109.2655	1748.24
5	logRB	0.2261	120.3963	1926.34
6	W, J	0.1915	101.9779	407.91
7	Sz, J	0.1936	103.0944	412.37
8	$^1\chi$, J	0.1535	81.7526	327.01
9	J, logRB	0.1840	97.9878	391.95
10	W, Sz	0.1824	97.1241	388.49
11	W, $^1\chi$	0.2079	110.7037	442.81
12	Sz, $^1\chi$	0.2026	107.8779	431.51

Looking to the sample size (8 compounds) we can't go for triparametric regression analysis. Hence, like *E. coli* here also we have correlated topological indices with antibacterial activity against *K. pneumonae* and observed that here also correlation splits into two sub-classes. In Class-I we have Mannich bases 2, 7, 8 and 12, while the Mannich bases belonging to Class-II are 1, 6, 10 and 11. Hence, we have carried out regression for the Mannich bases belonging to these two sub-classes. The results have shown that the same bi-parametric regression contain $^1\chi$ and J yielded excellent results:

Class - I

$$\text{Activity against } K.\ pneumonae = 6.1398 + 0.1963\ (\pm 0.1073)\ ^1\chi - 3.9856\ (\pm 1.3799)\ J \quad (4.2.8)$$

$n = 4$, $Se = 0.1608$, $r = 0.9888$, $R^2_A = 0.9333$, $F = 22.0020$, $Q = 5.8041$

Class - II

$$\text{Activity against } K.\ pneumonae = -69.1430 + 2.8603\ (\pm 1.0172)\ ^1\chi - 35.4501\ (\pm 9.98853)\ J \quad (4.2.9)$$

$n = 4$, $Se = 2.6162$, $r = 0.9626$, $R^2_A = 0.7796$, $F = 6.3060$, $Q = 0.3679$

4.2.3.3. Antibacterial Activity against *B. subtilis*

We now discuss antibacterial activity of Mannich bases against *B. subtilis*. Looking to the sample size (three Mannich bases) we can only go for monoparametric regression. Table 4.2.13 shows that all the five topological indices give excellent results, however, Balaban index (J) is found slightly better for this purpose. The model based on this index is found as:

$$\text{Antibacterial activity against } B.\ subtilis = 864.3680 - 790.6098\ (\pm 92.2738)\ J \quad (4.2.10)$$

$n = 3$, $Se = 0.7163$, $R = -0.9942$, $F = 85.1030$, $Q = 1.3879$

Table 4.2.13: Regression Analysis and Quality of Correlations for Modeling Antibacterial Activity of Mannich Bases against *B. subtilis* as well as Considering Entire Molecular Graph

Model	*Topological Index*	*Se*	R^2_A	*R*	*F*	*Q*
1	W	1.2795	–	–0.9813	25.987	0.7669
2	Sz	2.1195	–	–0.9478	8.835	0.4472
3	$^1\chi$	1.6531	–	–0.9686	15.166	0.5859
4	J	0.7163	–	–0.9942	85.103	1.3879
5	logRB	1.2870	–	–0.9811	25.671	0.7623

The results recorded in Tables 4.2.14 and 4.2.15 are in favour of this model.

In all the models discussed above we observed that Balaban index (J) play a dominating role and that the best model is one containing $^1\chi$ and J indices. This means that first-order branching and extended connectivity are favourable for the exhibition of antibacterial activity against all the three bacteria.

Earlier we have stated that the variation of structure of the Mannich bases is due to the variation in R-values. Alternatively we can say that the variation in antibacterial activity of the Mannich bases is due to variation in R. Consequently, we have

Table 4.2.14: Found and Estimated Antibacterial Activity of Mannich Bases against *B. subtilis* Using Best Model Containing J Index as well as Considering Entire Molecular Graph

Compound No.	Found	Estimated	Residue	$(Residue)^2$
1	21.03	20.55	0.48	0.2304
2	19.23	19.76	–0.53	0.2809
4	12.14	12.09	0.05	0.0025

$\Sigma(Residue)^2 = 0.5131$

Table 4.2.15: PE, LSE, LOF Values Calculated for the Derived Models for Modeling Antibacterial Activity of Mannich Bases against *B. subtilis* as well as Considering Entire Molecular Graph

Model	Topological Index	PE	LSE	LOF
1	W	0.0142	1.6371	3.6834
2	Sz	0.0391	4.4921	10.1072
3	$^1\chi$	0.0238	2.7328	6.1488
4	J	0.0044	0.5131	1.1544
5	logRB	0.0143	1.6565	3.7271

undertaken QSAR study for the rooted graphs of the Mannich bases. That is, we have calculated the topological indices for R skeleton (structural unit) and used them for correlation analysis. The results obtained are given in Tables 4.2.16 to 4.2.25, and are discussed below.

4.2.4. QSAR Study Based on Rooted-Graphs of the Mannich Bases

For the reason mentioned earlier we have obtained correlation matrices separately for the three bacteria used (Table 4.2.16), which again show that no monoparametric models are possible for modeling the antibacterial activity against *E. coli* and *K. pneumonae* and that excellent results will be obtained for *B. subtilis*. This is confirmed from the data recorded in Tables 4.2.17 to 4.2.19. The results (Tables 4.2.16 to 4.2.25) did show that biparametric regression gave quite a good statistics for *E. coli* and *K. pneumonae*. In order to compare our results obtained from rooted graphs we have made regression analysis for the same separated classes and the results are discussed below.

4.2.4.1. QSAR Study against *E. coli* Considering Rooted Graphs

Class – I

$$\text{Antibacterial activity against } E.\ coli = 15.2090 - 0.2214\ (\pm\ 0.0890)\ {}^1\chi - 0.9554\ (\pm\ 0.6907)\ J \qquad (4.2.11)$$

$n = 5, Se = 0.4422, r = 0.8709, R^2_A = 0.5170, F = 3.141, Q = 1.9695$

Table 4.2.16: Correlation Matrix for the Calculation of Antibacterial Activity of Mannich Bases (Rooted graph)

	Activity	*W*	*Sz*	$^1\chi$	*J*	*logRB*
(A) For *E. coli*						
Activity	1.0000					
W	–0.1921	1.0000				
Sz	–0.1921	0.9989	1.0000			
$^1\chi$	–0.0549	0.8956	0.8948	1.0000		
J	–0.0638	–0.6323	–0.6418	–0.4814	1.0000	
logRB	–0.1533	0.9963	0.9949	0.9271	–0.6220	1.0000
(B) For *K. pneumonae*						
Activity	1.0000					
W	–0.2215	1.0000				
Sz	–0.2239	0.9995	1.0000			
$^1\chi$	–0.1442	0.9227	0.9213	1.0000		
J	0.4795	–0.7204	–0.7223	–0.5649	1.0000	
logRB	–0.2154	0.9977	0.9970	0.9447	–0.7154	1.0000
(C) For *B. subtilis*						
Activity	1.0000					
W	–0.9806	1.0000				
Sz	–0.9107	0.9740	1.0000			
$^1\chi$	–0.9549	0.9945	0.9923	1.0000		
J	0.9999	0.9778	0.9050	0.9507	1.0000	
logRB	–0.9802	1.0000	0.9744	0.9947	0.9774	1.0000

Class – II

$$\text{Antibacterial activity against } E.\ coli = 14.5040 + 0.1616\ (\pm\ 0.0754)\ ^1\chi - 1.1781\ (\pm\ 0.7315)\ J \quad (4.2.12)$$

$n = 7$, $Se = 0.5412$, $r = 0.8372$, $R^2_A = 0.5514$, $F = 4.688$, $Q = 1.5469$

Comparison of these results obtained from the complete graph indicates that in the former cases better results are obtained. This indicates that the exhibition of the antibacterial activity depends on the molecular structure as a whole and not only on R-skeleton. Also, that the variation in the activity is due to variation in R. Thus, we can conclude that the antibacterial activities of the Mannich bases is not due to the substitutes but is a global activity.

4.2.4.2. QSAR study against *K. pneumonae* Using Rooted Graphs

In this case also we have carried out QSAR analysis under the same sub-classes. The results are given below:

Table 4.2.17: Regression Analysis and Quality of Correlations for Modeling Antibacterial Activity of Mannich Bases against *E. coil* (Rooted graph)

Model	Topological Index	Se	R^2_A	R	F	Q
1	W	0.9423	–	–0.1921	0.3834	0.2038
2	Sz	0.9423	–	–0.1921	0.3833	0.2038
3	$^1\chi$	0.9587	–	–0.0549	0.0302	0.0572
4	J	0.9582	–	–0.0638	0.0409	0.0665
5	logRB	0.9488	–	–0.1533	0.2407	0.1615
6	W, J	0.9633	–0.1071	0.3056	0.4677	0.3172
7	Sz, J	0.9621	–0.1043	0.3106	0.4805	0.3228
8	$^1\chi$, J	1.0052	–0.2055	0.1167	0.0621	0.1160
9	J, logRB	0.9788	–0.1429	0.2546	0.3120	0.2601
10	W, Sz	0.9933	–0.1770	0.1922	0.1726	0.1935
11	W, $^1\chi$	0.9568	–0.0923	0.3260	0.5353	0.3407
12	Sz, $^1\chi$	0.9572	–0.0931	0.3249	0.5313	0.3394

Table 4.2.18: Regression Analysis and Quality of Correlations for Modeling Antibacterial Activity of Mannich Bases Against *K. pneumonae* (Rooted graph)

Model	Topological Index	Se	R^2_A	R	F	Q
1	W	4.4437	–	–0.2215	0.3097	0.0498
2	Sz	4.4412	–	–0.2239	0.3167	0.0504
3	$^1\chi$	4.5093	–	–0.1442	0.1275	0.0319
4	J	3.9988	–	0.4795	1.7916	0.1199
5	logRB	4.4499	–	–0.2154	0.2920	0.0484
6	W, J	4.2888	–0.333	0.5117	0.8869	0.1193
7	Sz, J	4.2904	–0.0342	0.5111	0.8843	0.1191
8	$^1\chi$, J	4.3130	–0.0451	0.5035	0.8489	0.1167
9	J, logRB	4.2846	–0.0313	0.5131	0.8935	0.1197
10	W, Sz	4.8498	–0.3214	0.2368	0.1486	0.0488
11	W, $^1\chi$	4.8050	–0.2971	0.2710	0.1982	0.0564
12	Sz, $^1\chi$	4.7995	–0.2942	0.2749	0.2044	0.0572

Class - I

Antibacterial activity against *K. pneumonae* = 14.4864 - 0.0991 (± 0.0706) $^1\chi$ + 0.2699 (± 0.9525) J (4.2.13)

n = 4, Se = 0.4704, r = 0.8999, R^2_A = 0.4300, F = 2.131, Q = 1.9130

Class - II

Antibacterial activity against *K. pneumonae* = -5.9567 + 0.7472 (± 2.6117) $^1\chi$ + 9.4828 (± 20.1799) J (4.2.14)

$n = 4, Se = 8.7314, r = 0.4262, R^2_A = 1.4549, F = 0.1110, Q = 0.0488$

We observed that very bad statistics is obtained in this case. Furthermore, the model for Class-II is not allowed statistical as the coefficients of both $^1\chi$ and J are very small compared to their standard deviations.

Table 4.2.19: Regression Analysis and Quality of Correlations for Modeling Antibacterial Activity of Mannich Bases against *B. subtilis* (Rooted graph)

Model	*Topological Index*	*Se*	R^2_A	*R*	*F*	*Q*
1	W	1.3030	–	–0.9806	25.0189	0.7525
2	Sz	2.7447	–	–0.9107	4.8646	0.3318
3	$^1\chi$	1.9740	–	–0.9549	10.3376	0.4837
4	J	0.0913	–	–0.9999	5288.93	10.95
5	logRB	1.3157	–	–0.9802	24.5223	0.7450

Regression analysis has shown that the best bi-parametric model for the sub-class I is the one contains W and Sz as the correlating parameters. This model is found as below:

Class - I

Antibacterial activity against *K. pneumonae* = 14.9584 - 0.0200 (± 0.0113) W + 0.0132 (± 0.0077) Sz (4.2.15)

$n = 4, Se = 0.3486, r = 0.9463, R^2_A = 0.6869, F = 4.2905, Q = 2.7145$

Same is found to be the case for the Mannich bases belonging to Class-II.

Class - II

Antibacterial activity against *K. pneumonae* = 16.3329 + 0.4653 (± 0.0784) W + 0.3016 (± 0.0509) Sz (4.2.16)

$n = 4, Se = 1.6038, r = 0.9861, R^2_A = 0.9177, F = 17.6091, Q = 0.6148$

These results, therefore, again show that the anti-bacterial activity of Mannich bases is a global property.

4.2.4.3. QSAR Study against *B. subtilis* Considering Rooted Graphs

We now discuss the results obtained for antibacterial activity of Mannich bases against *B. subtilis* considering rooted graphs. As stated earlier excellent results are obtained in each cases and that the Balaban index J is found better for this purpose. This model is given below:

Antibacterial activity against *B. subtilis* = 351.8579 – 180.0406 (± 2.2270)J (4.2.17)

$n = 3, R = -0.9999, Se = 0.0913, F = 5288.93$

The results once again show antibacterial activity being global property.

4.2.5. Predictive Power of the Model

It is well known that a model with excellent statistics need not be a model with excellent predictive power. We have, therefore, to investigate the predictive powers of the proposed models. The simplest parameter for this purpose is the quality factor Q[30,31]. The calculated values of this Q factor indicates that the discussed models have excellent predictive power also. Another way of discussing predictive power is to estimate the antibacterial activity and compare these with their observed values. The residue *i.e.* difference between observed and estimated activities will be indicative of predictive power. The lowest value of the residues are in favour of better predictive power. In cases using the entire molecular graphs such comparison is given in Tables 4.2.8, 4.2.11 and 4.2.14, while the same using rooted graphs are given in Tables 4.2.20–4.2.22. The data show that results (predictive power) obtained considering entire molecular graphs are better than those considering rooted graphs. Also, that the proposed models have excellent statistics as well as excellent predictive power.

Table 4.2.20: Found and Estimated Antibacterial Activity of Mannich Bases against *E. coli* Using Best Model Containing W, $^1\chi$ (Rooted graph)

Compound No.	*Found*	*Estimated*	*Residue*	*(Residue)^2*
1	13.38	12.68	0.70	0.4900
2	12.05	12.66	–0.61	0.3721
3	11.29	12.69	–1.40	1.96
4	13.28	12.57	0.71	0.5041
5	14.21	12.66	1.55	2.4025
6	13.07	12.65	0.42	0.1764
7	12.84	12.22	0.62	0.3844
8	12.28	12.36	–0.08	0.0064
9	11.73	12.75	–1.02	1.0404
10	11.70	12.50	–0.80	0.64
11	12.83	12.47	0.36	0.1296
12	11.31	11.68	–0.37	0.1369

$\Sigma(\text{Residue})^2 = 8.2400$

Table 4.2.21: Found and Estimated Antibacterial Activity of Mannich Bases against *K. pneumonae* Using Best Model Containing J, logRB (Rooted graph)

Compound No.	*Found*	*Estimated*	*Residue*	*(Residue)^2*
1	19.35	15.79	3.56	12.6736
2	13.85	15.86	–2.01	4.0401
6	14.56	19.07	–4.51	20.3401
7	14.70	13.18	1.52	2.3104
8	15.08	17.30	2.22	4.9284
10	25.68	19.26	6.42	41.2146
11	13.44	15.91	–2.47	6.1009
12	13.84	14.08	–0.24	0.0576

$\Sigma(\text{Residue})^2 = 91.7880$

Table 4.2.22: Found and Estimated Antibacterial Activity of Mannich Bases against *B. subtilis* Using Best Model Containing J (Rooted graph)

Compound No.	*Found*	*Estimated*	*Residue*	*(Residue)²*
1	21.03	21.08	–0.05	0.0025
2	19.23	19.16	0.07	0.0049
4	12.14	12.15	–0.01	0.0001

$\Sigma(\text{Residue})^2 = 0.0075$

4.2.6. Use of Other Statistical Parameters

In favour of our results we have calculated three important statistical parameters *viz.*, (i) probable error of the coefficient of correlation (PE); (ii) least-square error (LSE), and (iii) Friedman's lack of fit measure (LOF)[32–34]. These parameters are calculated using the following expressions:

$$PE = \frac{2}{3}\,\frac{1-r^2}{\sqrt{n}} \tag{4.2.18}$$

where,

r is coefficient of correlation and 'n' is the number of compounds used. It is recommended that if,

(1) r < PE, r *i.e.* correlation is not significant.

(2) r > PE, several times, at least three times greater, correlation is indicated; and

(3) r > 6PE, correlation is definitely good.

Similarly, LSE is calculated from the following expression:

$$LSE = \Sigma\,(y_{obs} - y_{cal})^2 \tag{4.2.19}$$

where, y_{obs} and y_{cal} are the observed and calculated activities.

Finally, LOF is calculated from:

$$LOF = \frac{LSE}{\{1-(c+d.p)/M\}^2} \tag{4.2.20}$$

where,

c is the number descriptor + 1; p is the number of independent parameters, M is the number of samples used, and d is the smoothing parameters which controls the bias in the scoring factor between equations with different number of term and was kept 1. The advantage of using LOF is that it doesn't decrease with increased number of descriptors and the lowest value is found for an equation with the optimum number of parameters. The values of these parameters considering the entire molecular graphs of Mannich bases are recorded in Tables 4.2.9, 4.2.12 and 4.2.15, while their values considering rooted graphs are presented in Tables 4.2.23 to 4.2.25. The results show that the models attempted are definitely good in respect to the quality of regression and predictive power.

Table 4.2.23: PE, LSE, LOF Values Calculated for the Derived Models for Modeling Antibacterial Activity of Mannich Bases against *E. coli* (Rooted graph)

Model	*Topological Index*	*PE*	*LSE*	*LOF*
1	W	0.1853	8.8797	319.67
2	Sz	0.1853	8.8798	319.67
3	$^1\chi$	0.1918	9.1924	330.92
4	J	0.1916	9.1826	330.57
5	logRB	0.1879	9.0035	324.12
6	W, J	0.1744	8.3521	75.17
7	Sz, J	0.1738	8.3307	74.97
8	$^1\chi$, J	0.1898	9.0946	81.85
9	J, logRB	0.1799	8.6224	77.60
10	W, Sz	0.1853	8.8796	79.91
11	W, $^1\chi$	0.1719	8.2400	74.16
12	Sz, $^1\chi$	0.1721	8.2465	74.21

Table 4.2.24: PE, LSE, LOF Values Calculated for the Derived Models for Modeling Antibacterial Activity of Mannich Bases against *K. pneumonae* (Rooted graph)

Model	*Topological Index*	*PE*	*LSE*	*LOF*
1	W	0.2241	118.47	1895.52
2	Sz	0.2238	118.35	1893.60
3	$^1\chi$	0.2308	122.00	1952.00
4	J	0.1814	95.94	1535.04
5	logRB	0.2247	118.81	1900.96
6	W, J	0.1739	91.96	367.84
7	Sz, J	0.1741	92.04	368.16
8	$^1\chi$, J	0.1759	93.01	372.04
9	J, logRB	0.1736	91.788	367.15
10	W, Sz	0.2224	117.60	470.40
11	W, $^1\chi$	0.2183	115.44	461.76
12	Sz, $^1\chi$	0.2178	115.17	460.68

Table 4.2.25: PE, LSE, LOF Values Calculated for the Derived Models for Modeling Antibacterial Activity of Mannich Bases against *B. subtilis* (Rooted graph)

Model	*Topological Index*	*PE*	*LSE*	*LOF*
1	W	0.0147	1.6980	3.8205
2	Sz	0.0656	7.5333	16.9499
3	$^1\chi$	0.0339	3.8967	8.7675
4	J	0.00007	0.0075	0.0168
5	LogRB	0.0150	1.7310	3.8947

Table 4.2.26: Characterization Data of Nicotinoyl-4-aminobenzamido-methyl Amines

Sl.No.	Compound	Mol. Formula	m.p. (°C)	Elemental Analysis Found (Calcd.) %		
				C	H	N
1.	Nicotinoyl-4-aminobenzamidomethyl-sulphadiazine	$C_{24}H_{21}N_7O_4S$	165	56.85 (57.25	3.80 4.17	18.98 19.48)
2.	Nicotinoyl-4-aminobenzamidomethyl-sulphamethoxazole	$C_{24}H_{22}N_6O_5S$	140-142	56.60 (56.81	3.98 4.34	16.15 16.60)
3.	Nicotinoyl-4-aminobenzamidomethyl-sulphaguanidine	$C_{21}H_{21}N_7O_4S$	125	53.45 (53.96	4.05 4.49	20.65 20.98)
4.	Nicotinoyl-4-aminobenzamidomethyl-sulphadimidine	$C_{26}H_{25}N_7O_4S$	98-100	58.25 (58.75	5.00 4.70	19.00 18.45)
5.	Nicotinoyl-4-aminobenzamidomethyl-sulphamethiazole	$C_{23}H_{21}N_7O_4S_2$	140	52.33 (52.70	4.50 4.01	18.38 18.73)
6.	Nicotinoyl-4-aminobenzamidomethyl-sulphanilamide	$C\text{-}_{20}H_{19}N_5O_4S$	138-140	56.88 (56.47	4.90 4.47	16.98 16.47)
7.	Nicotinoyl-4-aminobenzamidomethyl-dimethylamine	$C\text{-}_{16}H_{18}N_4O_2$	120	64.08 (64.42	5.80 6.04	18.30 18.79)
8.	Nicotinoyl-4-aminobenzamidomethyl-diethylamine	$C\text{-}_{18}H_{22}N_4O_2$	100	66.60 (66.25	7.03 6.74	17.51 17.17)
9.	Nicotinoyl-4-aminobenzamidomethyl-diphenylamine	$C\text{-}_{26}H_{22}N_4O_2$	100-102	73.51 (73.93	4.86 5.21	12.95 13.27)
10.	Nicotinoyl-4-aminobenzamidomethyl-diethanolamine	$C\text{-}_{16}H_{22}N_4O_4$	69-70	59.86 (60.33	5.80 6.14	15.19 15.64)
11.	Nicotinoyl-4-aminobenzamidomethyl-morpholine	$C\text{-}_{16}H_{20}N_4O_3$	110	63.90 (63.52	6.20 (5.88)	16.83 16.47)
12.	Nicotinoyl-4-aminobenzamidomethyl-piperazine	$C\text{-}_{32}H_{32}N_8O_4$	130-132	65.00 (64.86	4.24 5.40	18.70 18.91)

4.2.7. Conclusion

From the above results we conclude that the newly synthesized Mannich bases are well characterized by ir and nmr data. Also, that the synthesized Mannich bases are activating only against three bacteria. Considering the results obtained from the entire molecular graphs as well as rooted graphs of Mannich bases indicate that the antibacterial activity is a global property and is not controlled solely by R and that variation in the activity is due to variation in R-skeleton.

4.3. Modeling of Antibacterial Activity of *p*-nitro-benzoyl-4-Aminobenzamido-methyl Amines

4.3.1. Introduction

Here we discuss the modeling of antibacterial activity of P-nitrobenzoyl-4-aminobenzamido-methyl amines (Figure 4.3.1, Table 4.3.1).

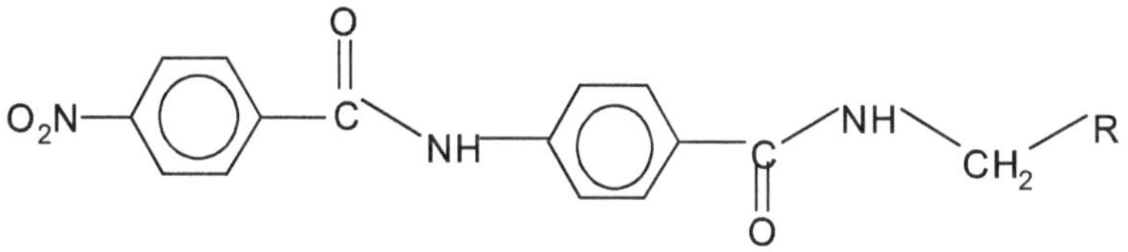

O_2N—(C₆H₄)—C(=O)—NH—(C₆H₄)—C(=O)—NH—CH_2—R

Figure 4.3.1: General Structures for the Newly Synthesis Mannich Bases

Here,

(1) R = —NH—(C₆H₄)—SO_2—NH—(pyrimidin-2-yl)

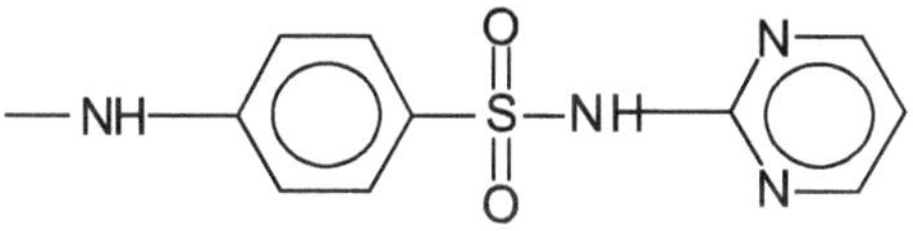

(2) R = —NH—(C₆H₄)—SO_2—NH—(5-methylisoxazol-3-yl, CH_3)

(3) R = —NH—(C₆H₄)—SO_2—NH—CH(NH_2)—NH_2

(4) R = —NH—(C₆H₄)—SO_2—NH—(4,6-dimethylpyrimidin-2-yl, CH_3, CH_3)

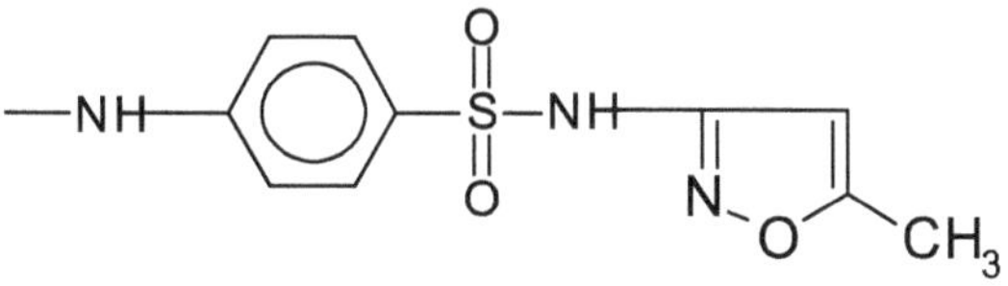

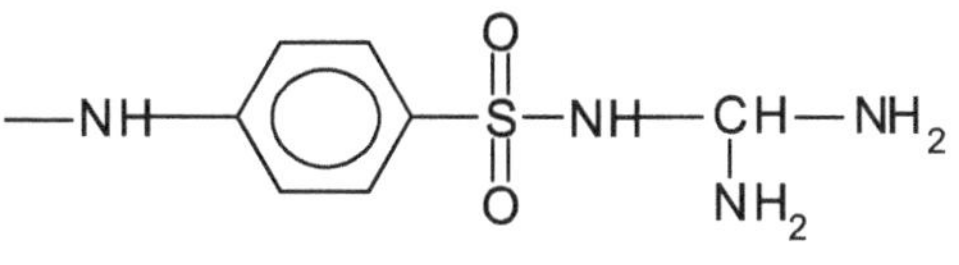

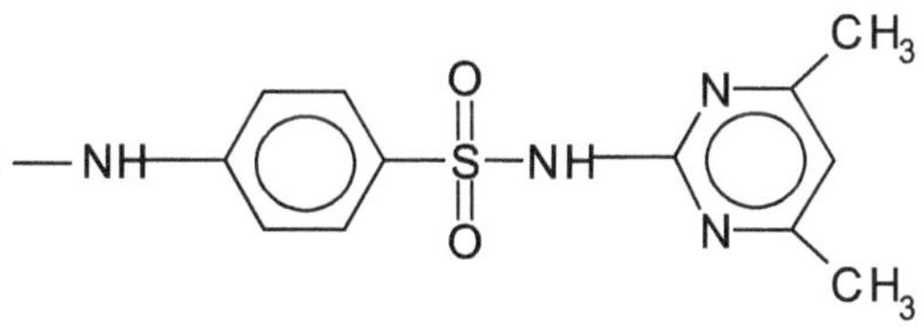

(5) R = —NH—(benzene ring)—SO_2—NH—(1,3,4-thiadiazole ring: S, N—N)—CH_3

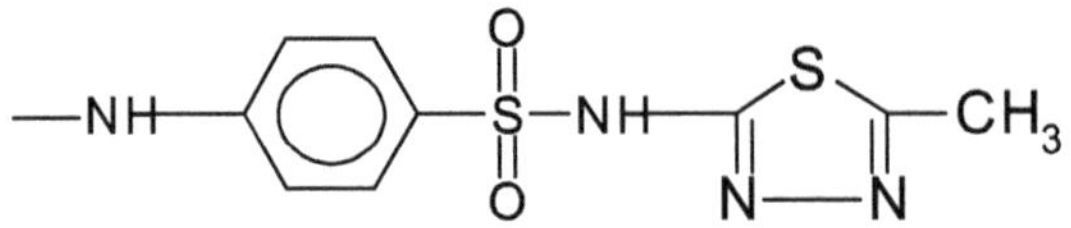

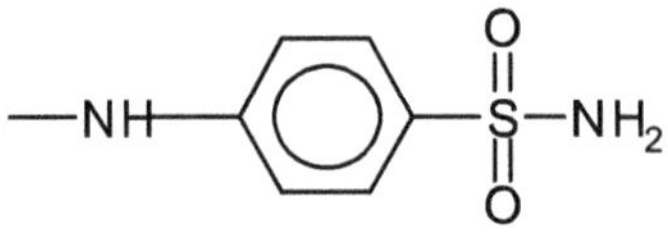

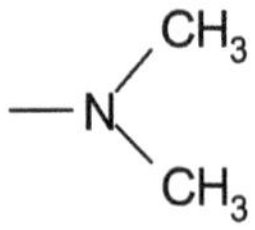

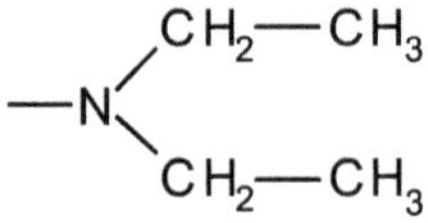

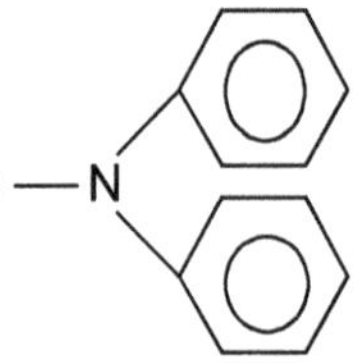

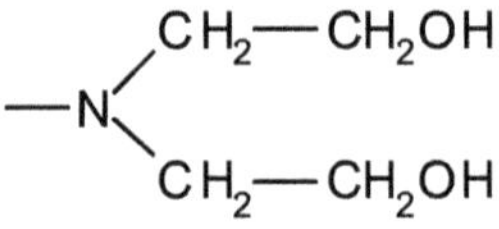

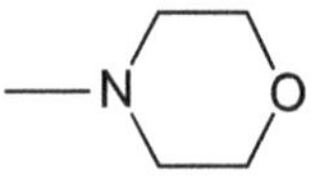

(6) R = —NH—(benzene ring)—SO_2—NH_2

(7) R = —N(CH_3)(CH_3)

(8) R = —N(CH_2—CH_3)(CH_2—CH_3)

(9) R = —N(benzene ring)(benzene ring)

(10) R = —N(CH_2—CH_2OH)(CH_2—CH_2OH)

(11) R = —N(ring)O

(12) R = —N(ring)N—CH_2—NH—C(=O)—(benzene ring)—NH—C(=O)—(benzene ring)—NO_2

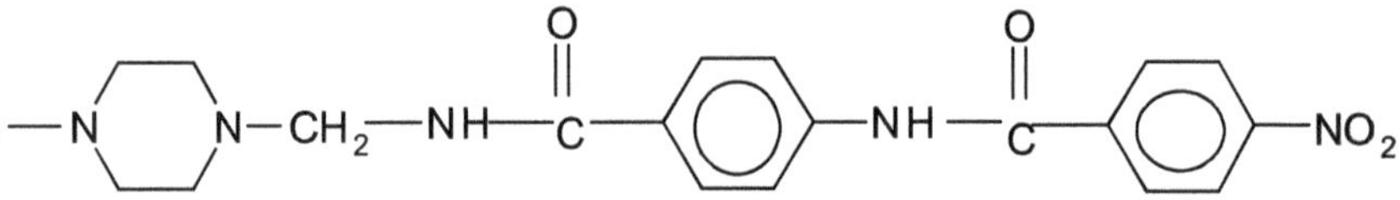

Like the earlier cases we have considered the R-skeleton as rooted graphs (Table 4.3.2). Hence, we have discussed modeling of antibacterial activity of these compounds under two different headings: (i) considering the entire molecular graphs and (ii) considering rooted graphs.

4.3.2. Results and Discussion

4.3.2.1. Characterization of Mannich bases

It is worthy to mention that here we have issued the compounds and Mannich bases as reported by Khosla in her Ph.D. Thesis. Hence, their characterization by elemental analysis, ir and nmr are given in Tables 4.3.3 to 4.3.5 and the antibacterial

Table 4.3.1: Name of the Mannich Bases along with their Molecular Structures: p-Nitrobenzoyl-4-Aminobenzamido-Methyl Amines

1. p-Nitrobenzoyl-4-Aminobenzamido-Methyl Sulphadiazine

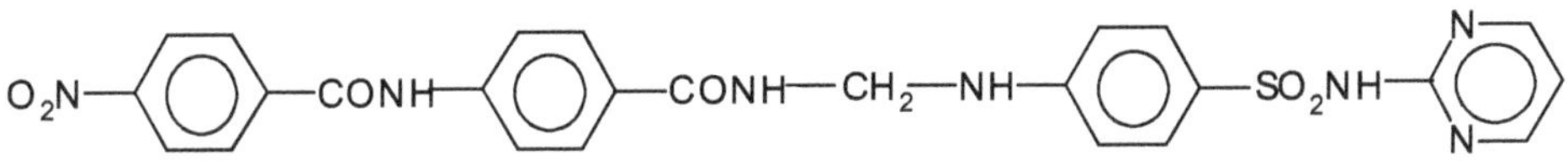

2. p-Nitrobenzoyl-4-Aminobenzamido-Methyl Sulphamethoxazole

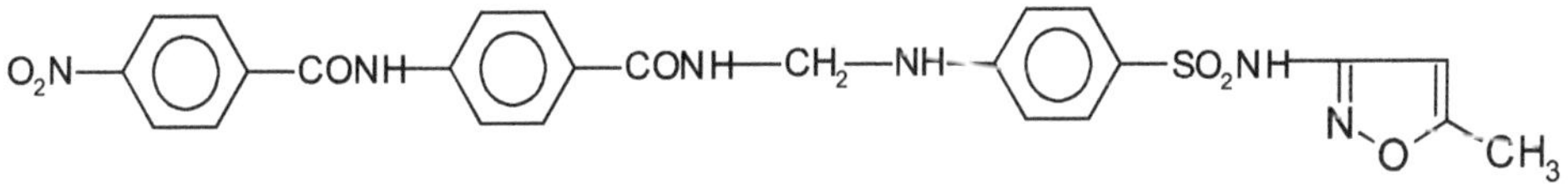

3. p-Nitrobenzoyl-4-Aminobenzamido-Methyl Sulphaguanidine

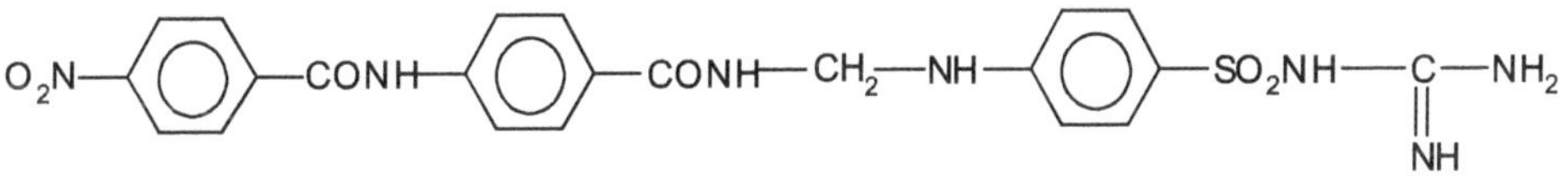

4. p-Nitrobenzoyl-4-Aminobenzamido-Methyl Sulphadimidine

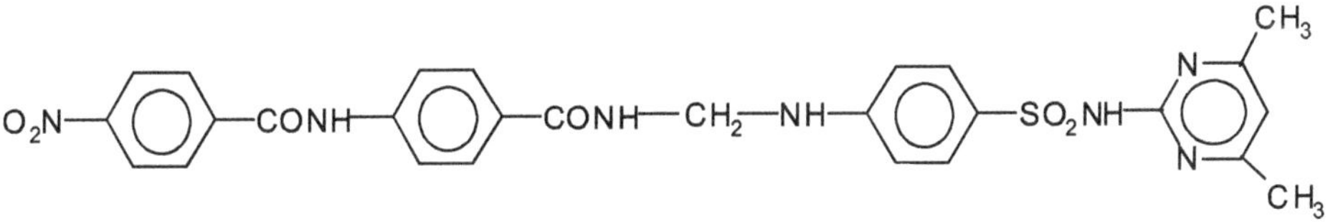

5. p-Nitrobenzoyl-4-Aminobenzamido-Methyl Sulphamethiazole

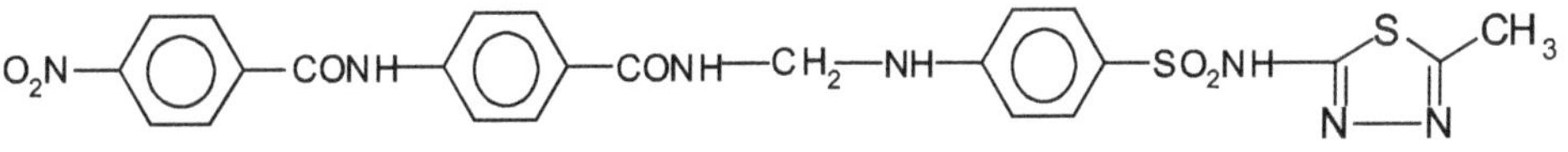

6. p-Nitrobenzoyl-4-Aminobenzamido-Methyl Sulphanilamide

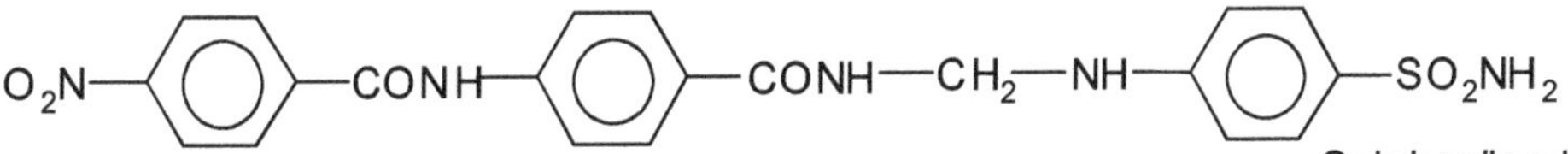

Sulphanilamide

7. p-Nitrobenzoyl-4-Aminobenzamido-Methyl

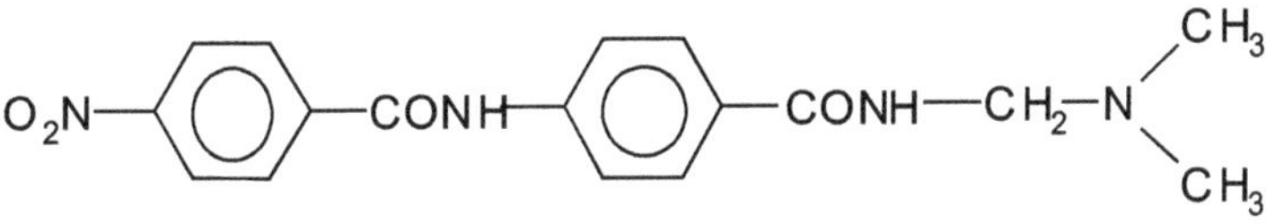

8. p-Nitrobenzoyl-4-Aminobenzamido-Methyl Diethyl amine

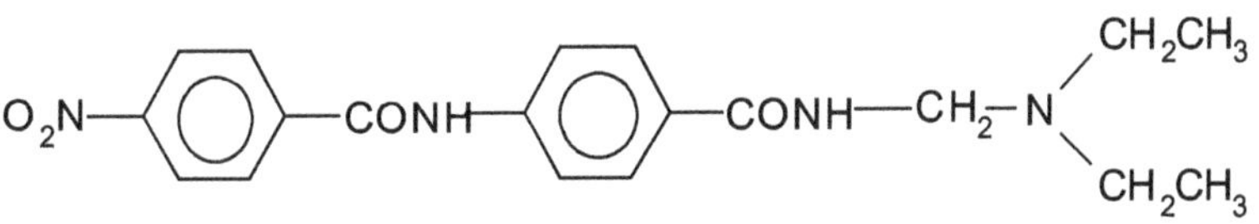

Contd...

Table 4.3.1–*Contd...*

9. p-Nitrobenzoyl-4-Aminobenzamido-Methyl Diphenyl amine

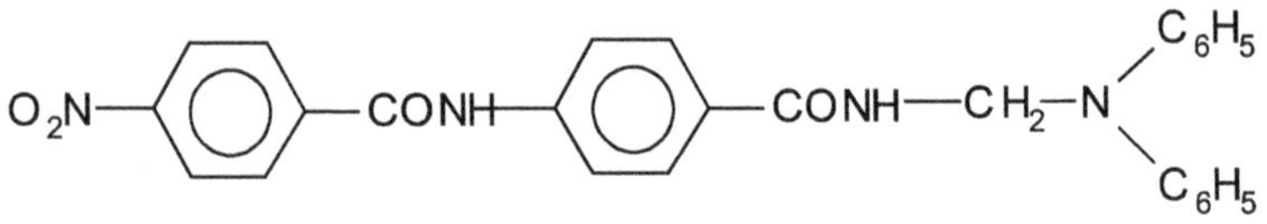

$O_2N-C_6H_4-CONH-C_6H_4-CONH-CH_2-N(C_6H_5)_2$

10. p-Nitrobenzoyl-4-Aminobenzamido-Methyl Diethanol amine

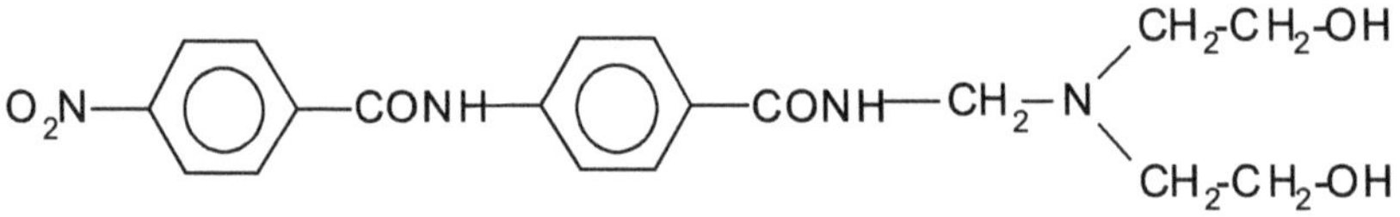

$O_2N-C_6H_4-CONH-C_6H_4-CONH-CH_2-N(CH_2\text{-}CH_2\text{-}OH)_2$

11. p-Nitrobenzoyl-4-Aminobenzamido-Methyl Morpholine

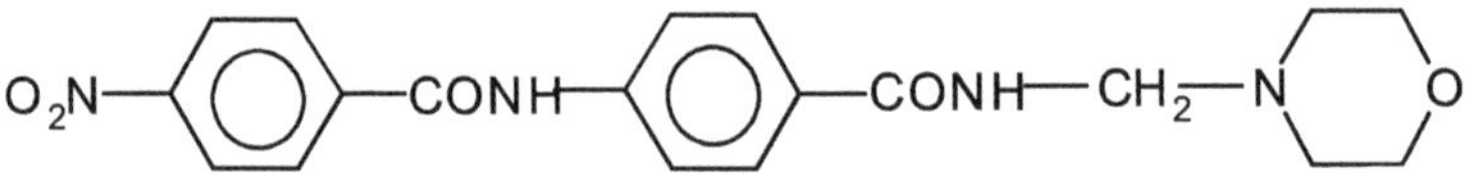

$O_2N-C_6H_4-CONH-C_6H_4-CONH-CH_2-N$ (morpholine ring, O)

12. Bis-p-Nitrobenzoyl-4-aminobenzamido methyl piperazine

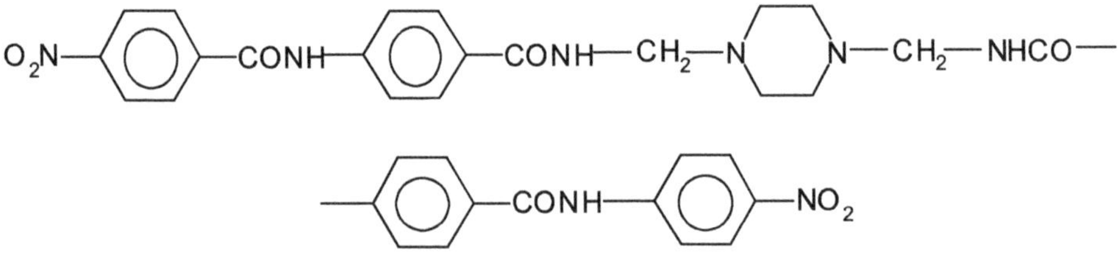

$O_2N-C_6H_4-CONH-C_6H_4-CONH-CH_2-N$ (piperazine ring) $N-CH_2-NHCO-$

$-C_6H_4-CONH-C_6H_4-NO_2$

Table 4.3.2: Structure of Rooted Graphs of Mannich Bases: p-Nitrobenzoyl-4-Aminobenzamido-Methyl Amines

General Structure:

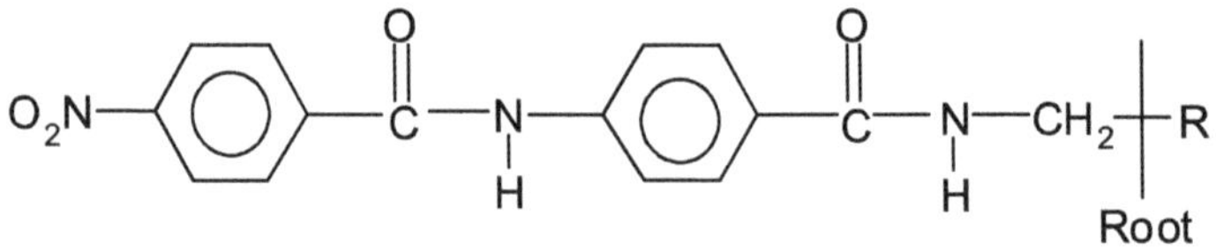

$O_2N-C_6H_4-C(=O)-NH-C_6H_4-C(=O)-NH-CH_2-R$ (Root)

R =

(1) $-NH-C_6H_4-SO_2-NH-$ (pyrimidin-2-yl)

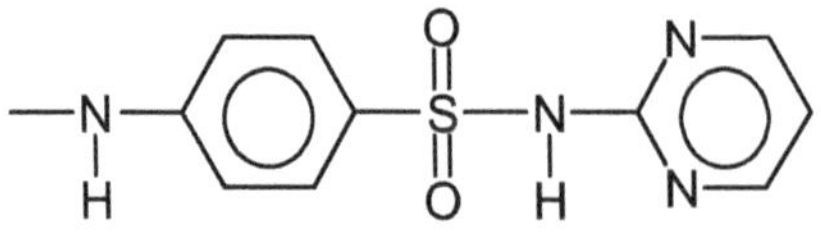

Contd...

Table 4.3.2–*Contd...*

(2)

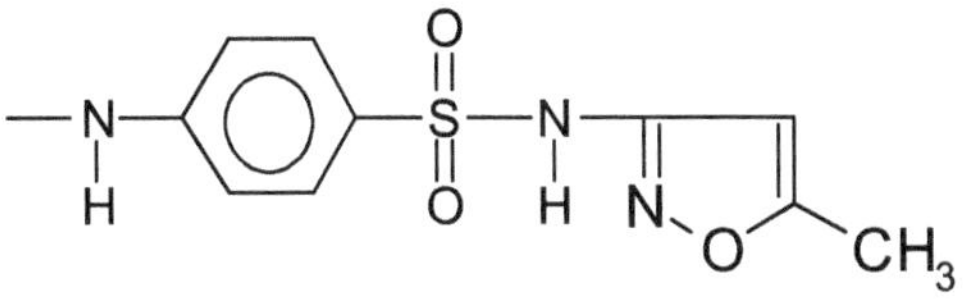

(3)

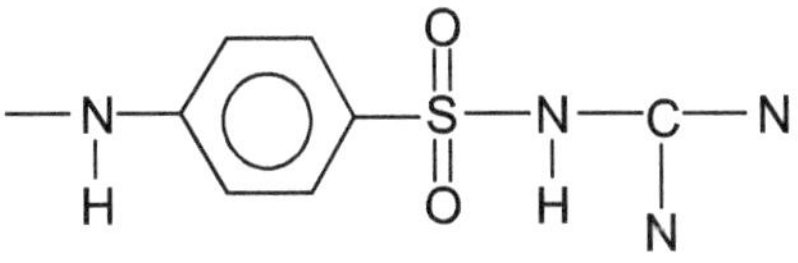

(4)

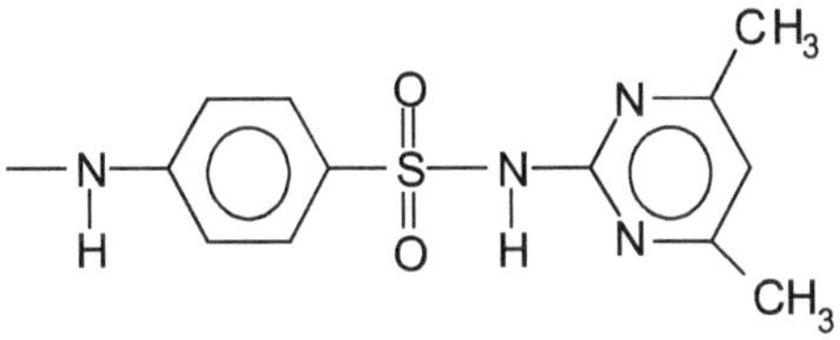

(5)

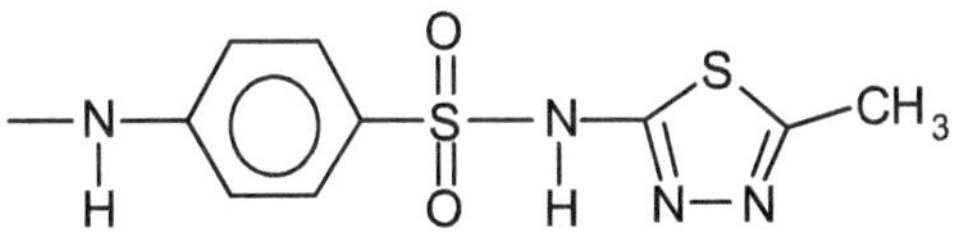

(6)

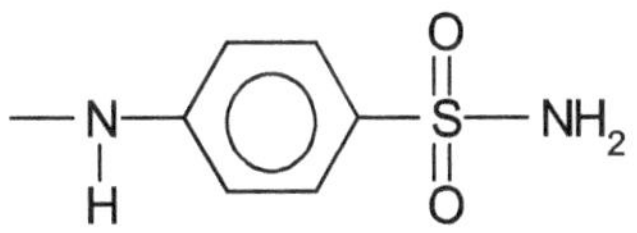

(7)

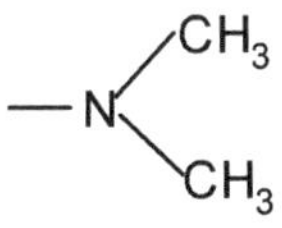

(8)

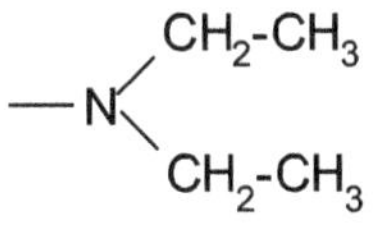

(9)

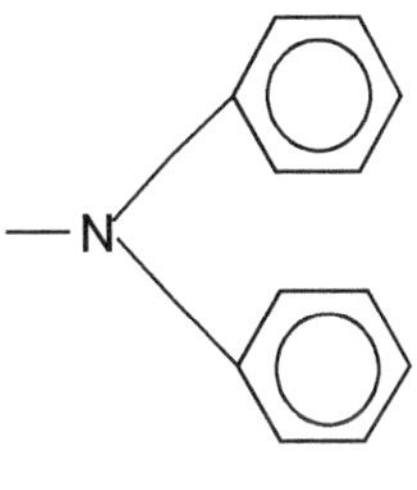

(10)

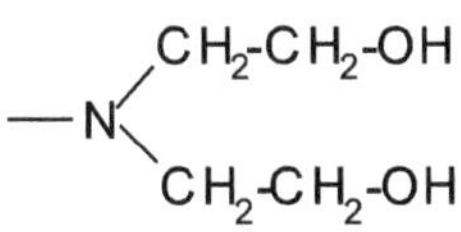

Contd...

Table 4.3.2–*Contd...*

(11)	—N O (morpholine ring)
(12)	—N N—CH_2—N(H)—C(=O)—⟨◯⟩—N(H)—C(=O)—⟨◯⟩—NO_2

activity are presented in Table 4.3.6. This table shows that out of the 12 newly synthesized Mannich bases of this series, only six (3,4,6,7,8,10) are active against *E. coli*, seven (1,2,3,5,6,8,9) are active against *K. pneumonae* and seven (1,2,3,4,5,7,8) against *B. subtilis*. Also, that different Mannich bases are active in each case; while Mannich bases 3 and 8 are active against all three bacteria used.

A perusal of Table 4.3.6 gives the following sequence for the anti-bacterial activity:

E. coli

$$6 > 3 > 10 > 8 > 7 > 4 \qquad (4.3.1)$$

K. pneumonea

$$3 > 9 > 1 > 8 > 2 > 5 > 6 \qquad (4.3.2)$$

B. subtilis

$$2 > 1 > 4 > 3 > 5 > 7 > 8 \qquad (4.3.3)$$

Obviously, same sequence exhibits in case of rooted graphs. However, this sequence doesn't give any structural activity relationship.

4.3.3. Structure-Activity Relationship Considering Entire Molecular Graph

In view of the above we have used topological indices, W, Sz, ${}^1\chi$, J and logRB in obtaining structural activity relationship. These indices calculated for the entire graphs of the Mannich bases are given in Table 4.3.7. Inspite of the fact that the topological indices used are very much susceptible for exhibiting degeneracy, no degeneracy is observed in any of the topological indices used.

In order to carry out modeling of antibacterial activity one has to obtain a correlation matrix. Since, different Mannich bases are found activity against the bacteria used, we have obtained three correlation matrices as shown in Table 4.3.8. These matrices show that none of the topological indices used are capable of modeling antibacterial activity against both the bacteria *i.e.*, *E. coli* and *K. pneumonae*. However, all the topological indices are useful for modeling the activity against *B. subtilis*, Szeged index Sz being slightly better for this purpose.

Table 4.3.3: Characterization Data of p-Nitrobenzoyl-4-aminobenzamido-methyl Amines

Sl.No.	*Compound*	*Mol. Formula*	*m.p. (°C)*	*Elemental Analysis Found (Calcd.) %*		
				C	*H*	*N*
1.	p-Nitrobenzoyl-4-aminobenzamido-methyl sulphadiazine	$C_{25}H_{21}N_7O_6S$	98-100	54.36 (54.84	3.49 3.83	17.60 17.91)
2.	p-Nitrobenzoyl-4-aminobenzamidomethyl-sulphamethoxazole	$C_{24}H_{22}N_6O_5S$	148	54.91 (54.54	4.50 4.00	15.64 15.27)
3.	p-Nitrobenzoyl-4-aminobenzamidomethyl-sulphaguanidine	$C_{22}H_{21}N_7O_6S$	150	51.30 (51.66	3.76 4.19	18.70 19.17)
4.	p-Nitrobenzoyl-4-aminobenzamidomethyl-sulphadimidine	$C_{27}H_{25}N_7O_6S$	152	56.81 (56.34	4.73 4.34	17.50 17.04)
5.	p-Nitrobenzoyl-4-aminobenzamidomethyl-sulphamethiazole	$C_{24}H_{21}N_7O_6S_2$	210	50.30 (50.79	3.40 3.70	16.90 17.28)
6.	p-Nitrobenzoyl-4-aminobenzamidomethyl-sulphanilamide	$C\text{-}_{21}H_{19}N_5O_6S$	168	53.45 (53.73	3.80 4.05	14.58 14.92)
7.	p-Nitrobenzoyl-4-aminobenzamidomethyl-dimethylamine	$C\text{-}_{17}H_{18}N_4O_4$	140-142	60.01 (59.64	5.64 5.26	16.83 16.37)
8.	p-Nitrobenzoyl-4-aminobenzamidomethyl-diethylamine	$C\text{-}_{19}H_{22}N_4O_4$	138-140	61.16 (61.62	5.36 5.94	14.76 15.13)
9.	p-Nitrobenzoyl-4-aminobenzamidomethyl-diphenylamine	$C\text{-}_{27}H_{22}N_4O_4$	180	69.18 (69.52	4.28 4.72	11.76 12.01)
10.	p-Nitrobenzoyl-4-aminobenzamidomethyl-diethanolamine	$C\text{-}_{19}H_{22}N_4O_6S$	158-160	56.46 (56.71	5.01 5.47	13.55 13.93)
11.	p-Nitrobenzoyl-4-aminobenzamidomethyl-morpholine	$C\text{-}_{19}H_{20}N_4O_5$	178	58.92 (59.37	4.83 5.20	14.06 14.58)
12.	p-Nitrobenzoyl-4-aminobenzamidomethyl-piperazine	$C\text{-}_{34}H_{32}N_8O_8$	175	59.60 (60.00	4.30 4.70	16.08 16.47)

Table 4.3.4: Ir Frequency Bands of P-nitrobenzoyl-4-aminobenzamido Methyl Amines

I	*II*	*III*	*IV*	*V*	*VI*	*VII*	*VIII*	*IX*	*X*	*XI*	*XII*
3398(s)	3500(m)	3420(s)	3395(s)	3420(m)	3420(m)	3320(s)	3400(m)	3420(w)	3350(m)	3500(w)	3420(m)
3110(s)	3400(s)	3350(s)	3125(s)	2910(w)	3300(w)	3200(m)	2970(m)	3100(m)	1660(s)	3400(m)	3350(m)
3040(m)	3120(s)	3195(s)	3048(s)	2840(w)	3049(w)	3100(m)	2810	3000(w)	1600	3125(m)	3220(m)
2940(m)	2915(w)	3010(w)	2950(w)	1675(m)	2940(w)	3005(m)	1670(s)	2940(w)	1520(m)	3025(m)	3000(s)
2850(m)	2850(m)	2920(w)	2901(w)	1600(s)	2800(w)	2950(w)	1600(s)	2790(w)	1450(s)	2940(w)	2925(w)
2800(m)	2798(w)	2800(w)	2790(w)	1510(s)	1670(s)	2770(m)	1510(s)	1670(m)	1350(s)	2800(m)	2810
2720(w)	1675(m)	1680(m)	1675(m)	1457(w)	1600(s)	1670(m)	1430(m)	1600	1315(w)	1678(m)	2749
1675(s)	1595(s)	1620(s)	1625(sh)	1430(m)	1520(s)	1600(s)	1400(m)	1510(m)	1250(m)	1600(s)	1660(m)
1650(w)	1510(s)	1575(sh)	1595(s)	1409(m)	1452(w)	1570(s)	1344(s)	1435(w)	1175(m)	1519(s)	1600(s)
1595(s)	1465(s)	1525(s)	1515(s)	1345(s)	1409(s)	1530(s)	1315(m)	1400(s)	1070(s)	1490(sh)	1630(w)
1580(sh)	1401(s)	1455(w)	1440(w)	1315(s)	1341(m)	1460(m)	1245(s)	1342(m)	1030(sh)	1459(w)	1520(s)
1510(s)	1345(s)	1402(s)	1402(s)	1290(m)	1320(m)	1405(m)	1175(s)	1310(m)	915(m)	1402(s)	1440(s)
1490(sh)	1260(s)	1342(s)	1382(sh)	1250(m)	1250(m)	1382(m)	1119(m)	1285(m)	850(w)	1345(s)	1460(sh)
1460(sh)	1160(s)	1310(m)	1310(s)	1175(s)	1175(sh)	1310(m)	1098(m)	1242(s)	785(m)	1315(s)	1375(s)
1440(s)	1090(s)	1260(m)	1260(m)	1090(m)	1149(s)	1260(w)	1020(m)	1181(s)	720(s)	1290(w)	1345(m)
1410(s)	1030(s)	1240(m)	1175(sh)	1010(w)	1090(s)	1240(m)	940(w)	1150(s)	665(w)	1265(w)	1312(m)
1370(sh)	1005(s)	1175(s)	1150(s)	1135(m)	1010(m)	1170(s)	870(s)	1040(w)		1247(w)	1255(m)
1325(s)	925(s)	1085(s)	1080(s)	895(w)	900(w)	1075(s)	853(s)	1010(w)		1175(s)	1172(s)
1260(s)	870(m)	1050(w)	1030(m)	875(w)	870(m)	1015(w)	772(s)	595(s)		1110(m)	1089(s)
1152(s)	855(w)	1009(w)	1005	851(m)	830(m)	920(s)	710(s)	870(s)		1011(s)	1060(s)
1095(s)	825(s)	1130(s)	975(m)	822(w)	760(s)	850(m)	690(w)	851(m)		870(s)	1010(s)
1040(w)	770(m)	940(w)	855(m)	770(s)	710(s)	790(m)	670(w)	769(s)		850(s)	950(s)

Contd...

Table 4.3.4–Contd...

I	II	III	IV	V	VI	VII	VIII	IX	X	XI	XII
1000(m)	712(s)	820(s)	825(m)	710(s)	650(w)	775(s)		710(m)		770(s)	895(w)
941(s)	680(m)	770(w)	771(s)	685(w)		720(s)		687(w)		749(w)	870(s)
870(w)		675(m)	724(s)			690(w)		669(w)		720(m)	770(s)
828(m)			675(s)			670(w)				690(s)	752(w)
799(s)										669(s)	710(m)
770(m)											665(m)
710(s)											
675(m)											

(m) = medium, (s) = strong, (w) = weak, (sh) = shoulder.

Table 4.3.5: ^1H NMR Spectral Data of p-Nitrobenzoyl-4-aminobenzene Amidomethyl Amines

Compd. No.	δ values in ppm					
	CH_2 (d)	NH (s)	Various (m) Ring Protons	CONH of Ring I (s)	CONH of Ring II (t)	SO_2NH (s)
I	2.82	6.1	6.5 – 8.01	7.9	8.33	10.6
II	2.90	6.08	6.6 – 8.01	8.1	8.3	10.9
III	3.05	5.90	6.65 – 8.0	7.9	8.2	10.7
IV	2.8	6.0	6.6 – 7.98	8.1	8.22	11.0
V	2.5	5.9	6.8 – 7.98	8.0	8.28	10.6
VI	2.55	6.1	6.7 – 7.8	8.0	8.3	10.95
VII	2.85	–	6.6 – 7.9	8.01	8.3	–
VIII	2.9	–	6.5 – 8.08.1	8.1	8.33	–
IX	2.9	–	6.6 – 8.1	7.9	8.2	–
X	2.5	–	7.75 – 8.08	7.9	8.31	–
XI	2.81	–	6.6 – 7.98	8.1	8.3	–
XII	2.79	–	6.6 – 7.7	7.9	8.3	–

(d) = doublet; (s) = singlet; (m) = multiplet; (t) = triplet.

Table 4.3.6: Antibacterial Activity of Mannich Bases

Compound No.	Zone of Inhibition in mm				Average
	Concentration in μg/ml				
	10	20	40	80	
(A) Against *E. coli*					
3	17.33	17.80	20.40	22.86	19.60
4	6.00	6.00	6.00	9.93	6.98
6	16.86	21.03	22.76	19.60	20.06
7	11.90	12.13	12.53	13.96	12.63
8	11.56	12.40	13.26	13.66	12.72
10	13.20	13.63	20.63	22.60	17.51
(B) Against *K. pneumonae*					
1	15.16	15.56	16.56	17.13	16.10
2	14.50	12.50	12.56	12.30	12.96
3	17.73	17.90	18.06	18.50	18.05
5	6.00	11.86	14.10	15.23	11.80
6	10.93	12.20	11.00	12.53	11.66
8	12.86	13.36	13.80	16.23	14.06
9	17.53	17.26	16.90	19.40	17.77

Contd...

Table 4.3.6–*Contd...*

Compound No.	*Zone of Inhibition in mm*				*Average*
	Concentration in μg/ml				
	10	*20*	*40*	*80*	
(C) Against *B. subtilis*					
1	15.80	13.23	21.20	21.96	18.05
2	12.80	17.86	20.26	21.50	18.10
3	8.76	10.03	16.23	18.23	13.31
4	8.63	17.43	20.46	19.76	16.57
5	8.16	11.40	11.43	11.93	10.73
7	8.90	9.20	9.80	10.06	9.49
8	9.03	9.50	9.60	9.76	9.47

Table 4.3.7: Distance Based Topological Indices Calculated for Mannich bases: P-Nitrobenzoyl-4-aminobenzimido-methyl Amines

Compound No.	*W*	*Sz*	$^1\chi$	*J*	*logRB*
1	6840	9852	18.7083	1.0603	1437.1820
2	6839	9633	18.6022	1.0611	1436.7760
3	5446	7711	17.0465	1.2677	1183.8820
4	7832	11278	19.4960	1.0692	1617.0900
5	6839	9633	18.6022	1.0611	1436.7760
6	4236	6078	15.6300	1.2677	955.4462
7	1832	2624	11.8631	1.6583	470.4000
8	2302	3220	12.9391	1.6509	573.6722
9	4538	6536	17.0080	1.7772	1061.7570
10	2836	3880	13.9391	1.6500	688.2968
11	2558	3764	13.5249	1.3094	627.0930
12	14593	22109	24.0497	0.87899	2662.6840

4.3.3.1. Modeling of Antibacterial Activity against *E. coli*

The results of regression analysis for modeling antibacterial activity against *E. coli* are shown in Table 4.3.9, which again show that none of the topological indices used singly are correlating with the activity. It means that no mono-parametric regression models are possible for modeling the activity against *E. coli*. However, the data did show that the Szeged index (Sz) will prove better in multiple regression analysis. Looking to the sample size (six Mannich bases) and in accordance with the "Rule of Thumbs" we can only go for biparametric regression analysis for modeling antibacterial activity of the Mannich bases against *E. coli*. Such analysis and the corresponding regression data are given in Table 4.3.9, which shows that a

Table 4.3.8 Correlation matrix for Mannich bases: P-Nitrobenzoyl-4-aminobenzimido-methyl amines

	Activity	*W*	*Sz*	*$^1\chi$*	*J*	*logRB*
(A) For *E. coli*						
Activity	1.0000					
W	–0.29184	1.0000				
Sz	–0.35452	0.98693	1.0000			
$^1\chi$	–0.33798	0.81084	0.88905	1.0000		
J	0.12751	–0.95111	–0.93240	–0.74070	1.0000	
logRB	–0.26771	0.99961	0.98557	0.81217	–0.95292	1.0000
(B) For *K. pneumonae*						
Activity	W	Sz	$^1\chi$	J	logRB	
Activity	1.0000					
W	–0.06043	1.0000				
Sz	–0.04502	0.99936	1.0000			
$^1\chi$	0.05504	0.97689	0.98038	1.0000		
J	0.03559	–0.93221	–0.93893	–0.97561	1.0000	
logRB	–0.02356	0.99765	0.99816	0.98917	–0.95047	1.0000
(C) For *B. subtilis*						
Activity	1.0000					
W	0.77483	1.0000				
Sz	0.78116	0.99962	1.0000			
$^1\chi$	0.77377	0.99711	0.99578	1.0000		
J	–0.77182	–0.98628	–0.98386	–0.98817	1.0000	
logRB	0.77400	0.99985	0.99925	0.99818	–0.98668	1.0000

biparametric model containing Sz and J is the correlating parameter is quite a good model:

$$\text{Antibacterial activity against } E.\ coli = 76.0813 - 0.0029\ (\pm 0.0023)\ Sz - 30.5309\ (\pm 20.9412)\ J \quad (4.3.4)$$

$n = 6$, $Se = 4.8856$, $R = 0.6643$, $R^2_A = 0.0688$, $F = 1.185$, $Q = 0.1359$

Plots of topological indices and the antibacterial activity against *E. coli* indicated that the data set (6 compounds) can be conveniently subdivided into two classes: (i) cotaining compounds 4,6,7, and (ii) containing compounds 3,8,10. When we attempted regression analysis under these two sub-classes, following best models are obtained:

(1) Subclass (i) Containing Mannich Bases 4,6,7

$$\text{Antibacterial activity against } E.\ coli = 18.5606 - 8.1 \times 10^{-4}\ (\pm 0.0127)\ Sz \quad (4.3.5)$$

$n = 3$, $Se = 7.8546$, $R = -0.4824$, $F = 0.3034$, $Q = 0.0614$

Table 4.3.9: Regression Analysis and Quality of Correlations for Modeling Antibacterial Activity of Mannich Bases against *E. coli*

Model	Topological Index	Se	R^2_A	R	F	Q
1	W	5.4139	–	–0.2918	0.372	0.0539
2	Sz	5.2927	–	–0.3545	0.575	0.0669
3	$^1\chi$	5.3273	–	–0.3380	0.516	0.0634
4	J	5.6141	–	0.1275	0.066	0.0227
5	logRB	5.4537	–	–0.2677	0.309	0.0491
6	W, J	5.3850	–0.1313	0.5667	0.710	0.1052
7	Sz, J	4.8856	0.0688	0.6643	1.185	0.1359
8	$^1\chi$, J	6.0342	–0.4206	0.3843	0.260	0.0636
9	J, logRB	5.6652	–0.2522	0.4987	0.497	0.0880
10	W, Sz	5.6396	–0.2409	0.5055	0.515	0.0896
11	W, $^1\chi$	6.1482	–0.4747	0.3393	0.195	0.0552
12	Sz, $^1\chi$	6.1028	–0.4531	0.3580	0.221	0.0587

However, this model is to be discarded as the coefficient of Sz term is quite smaller than its standard deviation. Such models are not allowed statistically.

(2) Subclass (ii) Containing Mannich Bases 3,8,10

Antibacterial activity against *E. coli* = -4.4233 + 1.4366 (± 0.8050) $^1\chi$ (4.3.6)

n = 3, Se = 2.4387, R = 0.8724, F = 3.1842, Q = 0.3577

The above results did show that improved correlation coefficients resulted by satisfying the data set into two sub-classes. However, such splitting doesn't always gives statistically significant results.

Table 4.3.10: Found and Estimated Antibacterial Activity of Mannich Bases against *E. coli* Using Best Model Containing Sz, J Indices

Compound No.	Observed Activity	Estimated Activity	Residue	$(Residue)^2$
3	19.60	14.842	4.758	22.6385
4	6.98	10.478	–3.498	12.2360
6	20.06	19.615	0.445	0.1980
7	12.63	17.783	–5.153	26.5534
8	12.72	12.416	0.304	0.0924
10	17.51	14.366	3.144	9.8847

$\Sigma(Residue)^2$ = 71.6058

Thus, using the best-model, without splitting we have estimated antibacterial activity against *E. coli* and compared them with the observed value. Such a comparison is shown in Table 4.3.10. The data presented in Table 4.3.10 are used to calculate PE, LSE and LOF (for details please see earlier reports). These parameters as given in

Table 4.3.11, show that all the models, including the one discussed here are quite good models having comparable predictive power.

Table 4.3.11: PE, LSE, LOF Values Calculated for the Derived Models for Modeling Antibacterial Activity of Mannich Bases against *E. coli*

Model	*Topological Index*	*PE*	*LSE*	*LOF*
1	W	0.2489	117.2425	1055.1826
2	Sz	0.2379	112.0500	1008.4501
3	$^1\chi$	0.2410	113.5186	1021.6675
4	J	0.2676	126.0739	1134.6652
5	logRB	0.2526	118.9731	1070.7589
6	W, J	0.1847	86.9932	195.7348
7	Sz, J	0.1520	71.6058	161.1130
8	$^1\chi$, J	0.2319	109.2351	245.7789
9	J, logRB	0.2044	96.2839	216.6388
10	W, Sz	0.2025	95.4153	214.6844
11	W, $^1\chi$	0.2407	113.4002	255.1504
12	Sz, $^1\chi$	0.2226	111.7325	251.3981

Table 4.3.12: Regression Analysis and Quality of Correlations for Modeling Antibacterial Activity of Mannich Bases against *K. pneumonae*

Model	*Topological Index*	*Se*	R^2_A	*R*	*F*	*Q*
1	W	2.9496	–	–0.0604	0.018	0.0205
2	Sz	2.9520	–	–0.0450	0.010	0.0152
3	$^1\chi$	2.9505	–	0.0550	0.015	0.0186
4	J	2.9531	–	0.0356	0.0063	0.0120
5	logRB	2.9542	–	–0.0236	0.0028	0.0080
6	W, J	3.2923	–0.4896	0.0833	0.014	0.0253
7	Sz, J	3.2998	–0.4964	0.0490	0.0048	0.0148
8	$^1\chi$, J	3.0126	–0.2472	0.4105	0.405	0.1362
9	J, logRB	3.2999	–0.4965	0.0486	0.0047	0.0147
10	W, Sz	2.9786	–0.2192	0.4327	0.461	0.1453
11	W, $^1\chi$	2.7867	–0.0672	0.5372	0.811	0.1928
12	Sz, $^1\chi$	2.8512	–0.1172	0.5052	0.685	0.1771

4.3.3.2. Modeling of Antibacterial Activity of Mannich bases against *K. pneumonae*

The regression parameters as well as quality of correlation the modeling antibacterial activity against *K. pneumonae* are given in Table 4.3.12. The results obtained here are poor and show that no statistically significant mono- and bi-parametric regression models are possible for modeling the activity of Mannich bases against this bacteria. However, the results did show that first-order connectivity index ($^1\chi$) is a good index for this purpose and the biparametric model contains $^1\chi$ and W gave better results:

$$\text{Antibacterial Activity against } K.\ pneumonae = -19.0624 - 0.0039\ W + 3.2120\ ^1\chi \quad (4.3.7)$$

n = 7, Se = 2.7867, R = 0.5372, F = 0.8110, Q = 0.1928

No improvement is observed by splitting data in sub-set.

We have used the above model and calculated the antibacterial activity, the comparison of which with the observed activity is shown in Table 4.3.13.

Table 4.3.13: Found and Estimated Antibacterial Activity of Mannich Bases against *K. pneumonae* Using Best Model having W and $^1\chi$ Indices

Compound No.	*Found*	*Estimated*	*Residue*	*(Residue)^2*
1	16.10	14.27	1.83	3.3489
2	12.96	13.93	–0.97	0.9409
3	18.05	14.39	3.66	13.3956
5	11.80	13.93	–2.13	4.5369
6	11.66	14.57	–2.91	8.4681
8	14.06	13.49	0.57	0.3249
9	17.77	17.81	–0.04	0.0016

$\Sigma(\text{Residue})^2 = 31.0626$

Table 4.3.14: PE, LSE, LOF Values Calculated for the Derived Models for Modeling Antibacterial Activity of Mannich Bases against *K. pneumonae*

Model	*Topological Index*	*PE*	*LSE*	*LOF*
1	W	0.2510	43.5010	532.9045
2	Sz	0.2514	43.5720	533.7743
3	$^1\chi$	0.2511	43.5282	533.2377
4	J	0.2516	43.6052	534.1810
5	logRB	0.2518	43.6362	534.5608
6	W, J	0.2502	43.3576	132.7829
7	Sz, J	0.2513	43.5556	133.3892
8	$^1\chi$, J	0.2095	36.3032	111.1787
9	J, logRB	0.2513	43.5576	133.3954
10	W, Sz	0.2047	35.4874	108.6803
11	W, $^1\chi$	0.1792	31.0626	95.1293
12	Sz, $^1\chi$	0.1876	32.5184	99.5877

Even though the proposed model is not statistically good we have calculated PE, LSE and LOF (Table 4.3.14), which further show that the model is not statistically good.

4.3.3.3. Modeling of antibacterial activity of the Mannich bases against *B. subtilis*

Modeling of antibacterial activity of the Mannich bases against *B. subtilis* the regression obtained thereby are presented in Table 4.3.15. Very encouraging results are obtained in this case. All the mono- and bi-parametric models attempted were found statistically significant. Here also the mono-parametric model based on Szeged index (Sz) gave better results:

$$\text{Antibacterial Activity against } B.\ subtilis = 6.8419 + 8.8643 \times 10^{-4} (\pm 3.16 \times 10^{-4})\ Sz \quad (4.3.8)$$

n = 7, Se = 2.6650, R = 0.7812, F = 7.8270, Q = 0.2931

Table 4.3.15: Regression Analysis and Quality of Correlation for Modeling Antibacterial Activity of Mannich Bases against *B. subtilis*

Model	*Topological Index*	*Se*	R^2_A	*R*	*F*	*Q*
1	W	2.6985	–	0.7748	7.511	0.2871
2	Sz	2.6650	–	0.7812	7.827	0.2931
3	$^1\chi$	2.7040	–	0.7738	7.460	0.2861
4	J	2.7141	–	–0.7718	7.367	0.2843
5	logRB	2.7028	–	0.7740	7.471	0.2863
6	W, J	3.0089	0.4037	0.7762	3.031	0.2579
7	Sz, J	2.9783	0.4158	0.7814	3.135	0.2623
8	$^1\chi$, J	3.0149	0.4014	0.7752	3.012	0.2571
9	J, logRB	3.0124	0.4024	0.7756	3.020	0.2575
10	W, Sz	2.7882	0.4880	0.8116	3.859	0.2911
11	W, $^1\chi$	3.0161	0.4009	0.7750	3.007	0.2569
12	Sz, $^1\chi$	2.9720	0.4183	0.7824	3.157	0.2632

The data presented in Table 4.3.15 shows that better results are obtained in bi-parametric regression and thus a bi-parametric model containing Sz and W gave the best model:

$$\text{Antibacterial activity against } B.\ subtilis = 7.3843 + 0.0100 (\pm 0.0120)\ Sz - 0.0131 (\pm 0.0173)\ W \quad (4.3.9)$$

n = 7, Se = 2.7882, R = 0.8116, F = 3.8594, Q = 0.2911

We have, therefore, used the model and calculated anti-bacterial activity and compared them with the observed activity (Table 4.3.16). The data so obtained are then used to calculate PE, LSE and LOF and presented them in Table 4.3.17, which are in favour of the proposed models.

Table 4.3.16: Found and Estimated Antibacterial Activity of Mannich bases against *B. subtilis* Using Best Model Containing W, Sz Indices

Compound No.	*Found*	*Estimated*	*Residue*	*(Residue)²*
1	18.05	16.55	1.50	2.25
2	18.10	14.38	3.72	13.8384
3	13.31	13.35	–0.04	0.0016
4	16.57	17.85	–1.28	1.6384
5	10.73	14.38	–3.65	13.3225
7	9.49	9.69	–0.2	0.04
8	9.47	9.51	–0.04	0.0016

$\Sigma(\text{Residue})^2 = 31.0971$

Table 4.3.17: PE, LSE, LOF Values Calculated for the Derived Models for Modeling Antibacterial Activity of Mannich Bases against *B. subtilis*

Model	*Topological Index*	*PE*	*LSE*	*LOF*
1	W	0.1007	36.4093	446.0284
2	Sz	0.0982	35.5120	435.0361
3	$^1\chi$	0.1011	36.5592	447.8647
4	J	0.1018	36.8329	451.2176
5	logRB	0.1010	36.5264	447.4629
6	W, J	0.1001	36.2149	110.9083
7	Sz, J	0.0981	35.4815	108.6623
8	$^1\chi$, J	0.1005	36.3578	111.3459
9	J, logRB	0.1003	36.2986	111.1646
10	W, Sz	0.0860	31.0971	95.2350
11	W, $^1\chi$	0.1006	36.3875	111.4369
12	Sz, $^1\chi$	0.0977	35.3308	108.2007

4.3.4. Modeling of Antibacterial Activity Considering Root Graphs of the Mannich Bases Used

We now discuss the modeling of antibacterial activity of the Mannich bases under study by considering them rooted graphs. Since the rooted graphs are for the substitution R, the results obtained from the rooted graphs can be used to discuss effect of substitution on the antibacterial activity of Mannich bases under study.

Topological Indices for the Rooted Graphs

All the five topological indices (W, Sz, $^1\chi$, J and logRB) are calculated for the rooted graphs and are recorded in Table 4.3.18. Here, we observed that little degeneracy is present in the topological indices used.

Table 4.3.18: Distance Based Topological Indices Calculated for Mannich bases (Rooted)

Compound No.	*W*	*Sz*	*$^{1}\chi$*	*J*	*logRB*
1	536	818	8.0773	1.8372	162.0572
2	535	731	7.9712	1.8479	161.6517
3	307	427	6.4155	2.4613	96.2437
4	722	1092	8.8650	1.8868	215.2262
5	535	731	7.9712	1.8479	161.6517
6	152	236	4.9990	2.3936	48.2757
7	4	4	1.4142	1.6330	0.6931
8	20	20	2.4142	2.1906	5.6630
9	264	444	6.4495	1.6872	81.3185
10	56	56	3.4142	2.4478	17.0297
11	27	54	3.0000	2.0000	7.4547
12	2558	3764	13.5249	1.3094	627.0936

Table 4.3.19: Correlation Matrix for the Calculation of Antibacterial Activity of Mannich Bases (Rooted graph)

	Activity	*W*	*Sz*	*$^{1}\chi$*	*J*	*logRB*
(A) For *E. coli*						
Activity	1.0000					
W	–0.4917	1.0000				
Sz	–0.5069	0.9991	1.0000			
$^{1}\chi$	–0.2047	0.9488	0.9427	1.0000		
J	0.7724	–0.1405	–0.1631	0.1589	1.0000	
logRB	–0.4705	0.9996	0.9983	0.9555	–0.1228	1.0000
(B) For *K. pneumonae*						
Activity	1.0000					
W	–0.0595	1.0000				
Sz	0.0126	0.9908	1.0000			
$^{1}\chi$	0.0609	0.9614	0.9731	1.0000		
J	–0.0476	–0.5662	–0.6120	–0.5399	1.0000	
logRB	–0.0498	0.9997	0.9910	0.9661	–0.5550	1.0000
(C) For *B. subtilis*						
Activity	1.0000					
W	0.7701	1.0000				
Sz	0.7831	0.9963	1.0000			
$^{1}\chi$	0.7746	0.9756	0.9635	1.0000		
J	–0.1083	–0.1639	–0.1732	–0.0047	1.0000	
logRB	0.7721	0.9997	0.9952	0.9797	–0.1503	1.0000

Correlation Matrices of the Rooted Graphs

Once again three different correlation matrices are obtained as different number of Mannich bases were found active against the bacteria used. These matrices are given in Table 4.3.19, which shows that the topological indices can be used successively for modeling antibacterial activity against *E. coli* and *B. subtilis*. However, the topological indices are not useful for modeling the antibacterial activity against *K. pneumonae*.

4.3.4.1. Modeling of Antibacterial Activity of Rooted Mannich Bases against *E. coli*

The regression parameters and quality of correlation for modeling antibacterial activity against *E. coli* under rooted condition are presented in Table 4.3.20, which shows that in rooted parametric modeling only J index resulted in the statistically significant result:

$$\text{Antibacterial activity Against } E.\ coli \text{ (rooted)} = -9.9633 + 11.4715\ (\pm 4.7164)\ J \qquad (4.3.10)$$

n = 6, Se = 3.5951, R = 0.7724, F = 5.9156, Q = 0.2148

Table 4.3.20: Regression Analysis and Quality of Correlation for Modeling Antibacterial Activity of Mannich Bases against *E. coli* (Rooted graph)

Model	*Topological Index*	*Se*	R^2_A	*R*	*F*	*Q*
1	W	4.9288	–	–0.4917	1.2754	0.0997
2	Sz	4.8792	–	–0.5069	1.3831	0.1039
3	$^1\chi$	5.5404	–	–0.2047	0.1750	0.0369
4	J	3.5951	–	0.7724	5.9156	0.2148
5	logRB	4.9944	–	–0.4705	1.1376	0.0942
6	W, J	3.2916	0.5773	0.8639	4.4140	0.2624
7	Sz, J	3.2963	0.5760	0.8635	4.3971	0.2619
8	$^1\chi$, J	3.5401	0.5110	0.8406	3.6128	0.2374
9	J, logRB	3.3333	0.5665	0.8601	4.2671	0.2580
10	W, Sz	5.1214	–0.0233	0.6213	0.9431	0.1213
11	W, $^1\chi$	1.7506	0.8804	0.9635	19.4088	0.5503
12	Sz, $^1\chi$	1.7614	0.8789	0.9630	19.1519	0.5467

The perusal of Table 4.3.20, shows that better results are obtained in bi-parametric regression analysis and that two bi-parametric models: (i) containing W, $^1\chi$ and (ii) Sz, $^1\chi$ gave excellent results. The bi-parametric model based on W and $^1\chi$ is found below:

$$\text{Antibacterial activity against } E.\ coli \text{ (rooted)} = 4.3630 - 0.0549\ (\pm 0.0090)W + 4.8174\ (\pm 0.8991)\ ^1\chi \qquad (4.3.11)$$

n = 6, Se = 1.7506, R = 0.9635, F = 19.4088, Q = 0.5503

The other biparametric model containing Sz and $^1\chi$ is found as:

$$\text{Antibacterial activity against } E.\ coli \text{ (rooted)} = 4.6867 - 0.0342\ (\pm 0.0056)\text{Sz} + 4.5094\ (\pm 0.8565)\ ^1\chi \quad (4.3.12)$$

n = 6, Se = 1.7614, R = 0.9630, F = 19.1519, Q = 0.5407

The statistics show that the former model is slightly better. We have, therefore, used the same and calculated the antibacterial activity and compared them with the observed ones (Table 4.3.21). The data presented in Table 4.3.21 are then used to calculate PE, LSE and LOF (Table 4.3.22), which are in favour of the proposed models.

Table 4.3.21: Found and estimated antibacterial activity of Mannich bases against *E. coli* using best model containing W, $^1\chi$ (Rooted graph)

Compound No.	*Found*	*Estimated*	*Residue*	*(Residue)^2*
3	19.60	18.41	1.19	1.4161
4	6.98	7.40	–0.42	0.1764
6	20.06	20.09	–0.03	0.0009
7	12.63	10.96	1.67	2.7889
8	12.72	14.89	–2.17	4.7089
10	17.51	17.74	–0.23	0.0529

Σ = 9.1340

Table 4.3.22 PE, LSE, LOF Values Calculated for the Derived Models for Modeling Antibacterial Activity of Mannich Bases against *E. coli* (Rooted graph)

Model	*Topological Index*	*PE*	*LSE*	*LOF*
1	W	0.2063	97.1728	874.55
2	Sz	0.2021	95.2292	857.06
3	$^1\chi$	0.2607	122.7853	1105.06
4	J	0.1097	51.6993	465.29
5	logRB	0.2118	99.7790	898.01
6	W, J	0.0690	32.5050	73.13
7	Sz, J	0.0691	32.5982	73.34
8	$^1\chi$, J	0.0798	37.5986	84.59
9	J, logRB	0.0780	33.3329	74.99
10	W, Sz	0.1670	78.6857	177.04
11	W, $^1\chi$	0.0195	9.1340	20.55
12	Sz, $^1\chi$	0.0197	9.3084	20.94

4.3.4.2. Antibacterial Activity of the Mannich Bases against *K. pneumonae* Considering the Rooted Graphs

The regression parameters for modeling antibacterial activity of rooted Mannich bases are presented in Table 4.3.23, which show that no statistically significant models are possible. However, a bi-parametric model containing W and Sz indices gave better results.

Table 4.3.23: Regression Analysis and Quality of Correlations for Modeling Antibacterial Activity of Mannich Bases against *K. pneumonae* (Rooted graph)

Model	*Topological Index*	*Se*	R^2_A	*R*	*F*	*Q*
1	W	2.9497	–	–0.0595	0.0177	0.0201
2	Sz	2.9547	–	0.0126	8×10^{-4}	0.0042
3	$^1\chi$	2.9495	–	0.0609	0.0186	0.0206
4	J	2.9516	–	–0.0476	0.0114	0.0161
5	logRB	2.9513	–	–0.0498	0.0124	0.0168
6	W, J	3.2817	–0.4800	0.1152	0.0269	0.0351
7	Sz, J	3.2993	–0.4959	0.0520	0.0054	0.0157
8	$^1\chi$, J	3.2971	–0.4939	0.0634	0.00807	0.0192
9	J, logRB	3.2861	–0.4839	0.1033	0.0216	0.0314
10	W, Sz	2.7915	–0.0709	0.5348	0.8013	0.1916
11	W, $^1\chi$	2.9764	–0.2174	0.3413	0.4642	0.1146
12	Sz, $^1\chi$	3.229	–0.4328	0.2116	0.0937	0.0655

Antibacterial activity against *K. pneumonae* (rooted) = 14.2453 – 0.0515 (± 0.0407) W + 0.0363 (± 0.0288) Sz (4.3.13)

n = 7, Se = 2.7915, R = 0.5348, F = 0.8013, Q = 0.1916

We have observed that when the data set is splitted under two subclasses: (i) containing compounds 1,6,9 and (ii) containing 2,3,5,8 compounds, better results are obtained.

Table 4.3.24: Found and Estimated Antibacterial Activity of Mannich bases against *K. pneumonae* Using Best Model Containing W, Sz (Rooted graph)

Compound No.	*Found*	*Estimated*	*Residue*	*(Residue)²*
1	16.10	16.33	–0.23	0.0529
2	12.96	13.23	–0.27	0.0729
3	18.05	13.93	4.12	16.9744
5	11.80	13.23	–1.43	2.0449
6	11.66	14.98	–3.32	11.0224
8	14.06	13.94	0.12	0.0144
9	17.77	16.78	0.99	0.9801

Σ = 31.1711

(1) Subclass (i) Containing Mannich Bases 1,6,9

$$\text{Antibacterial activity against } K.\ pneumonae \text{ (rooted)} = 31.8798 - 8.4673\,(\pm 0.5485)\,J \quad (4.3.14)$$

n = 3, Se = 0.2887, R = -0.9979, F = 238.3001, Q = 3.4566

(2) Subclass (ii) Containing Mannich Bases 2,3,5,8

$$\text{Antibacterial activity against } K.\ pneumonae \text{ (rooted)} = -3.8592 + 8.6619\,(\pm 2.0560)\,J \quad (4.3.15)$$

n = 4, Se = 1.0590, R = 0.9480, F = 17.7386, Q = 0.8951

The comparison of observed and estimated activity (Table 4.3.24) and the values of PE, LSE and LOF (Table 4.3.25) are in favour of proposed models.

Table 4.3.25: PE, LSE, LOF Values Calculated for the Derived Models for Modeling Antibacterial Activity of Mannich Bases against *K. pneumonae* (Rooted graph)

Model	*Topological Index*	*PE*	*LSE*	*LOF*
1	W	0.2510	43.5057	532.94
2	Sz	0.2519	43.6535	534.75
3	$^1\chi$	0.2510	43.4984	532.85
4	J	0.2513	43.5612	533.62
5	logRB	0.2513	43.5521	533.51
6	W, J	0.2486	43.0802	131.93
7	Sz, J	0.2513	43.5422	133.34
8	$^1\chi$, J	0.2509	43.4849	133.17
9	J, logRB	0.2493	43.1942	132.28
10	W, Sz	0.1798	31.1711	95.46
11	W, $^1\chi$	0.2226	35.4360	108.52
12	Sz, $^1\chi$	0.2406	41.7058	127.72

4.3.4.3. Antibacterial Activity of Mannich Bases against *B. subtilis* Considering Rooted Graphs

The regression data and quality of correlation for modeling antibacterial activity against *B. subtilis* considering rooted graphs of Mannich bases are presented in Table 4.3.26, which shows that all the models, except the one based on J index, are statistically significant. Among the mono-parametric models, the model based on Sz gave better results.

$$\text{Antibacterial activity against } B.\ subtilis \text{ (rooted)} = 9.6425 + 0.0074\,(\pm 0.0026)\,Sz \quad (4.3.16)$$

n = 7, Se = 2.6546, R = 0.7831, F = 7.9280, Q = 0.2950

The biparametric modeling slight improvements in the correlation coefficient (R) are observed in that it is found highest for model containing W and Sz indices:

Antibacterial activity against *B. subtilis* (rooted) = 9.8926 – 0.0190 (± 0.0496)W + 0.0202 (± 0.0334) Sz (4.3.17)

n = 7, Se = 2.9148, R = 0.7918, F = 3.3614, Q = 0.2716

Table 4.3.26: Regression Analysis and Quality of Correlations for Modeling Antibacterial Activity of Mannich Bases against *B. subtilis* (Rooted graph)

Model	*Topological Index*	*Se*	R^2_A	*R*	*F*	*Q*
1	W	2.7229	–	0.7701	7.2872	0.2828
2	Sz	2.6546	–	0.7831	7.9280	0.2950
3	$^1\chi$	2.6996	–	0.7746	7.5009	0.2869
4	J	4.2434	–	–0.1083	0.0594	0.0255
5	logRB	2.7126	–	0.7721	7.3808	0.2846
6	W, J	3.0431	0.3901	0.7703	2.9188	0.2531
7	Sz, J	2.9650	0.4210	0.7836	3.1815	0.2642
8	$^1\chi$, J	2.9765	0.4165	0.7816	3.1414	0.2626
9	J, logRB	3.0326	0.3943	0.7721	2.9531	0.2546
10	W, Sz	2.9148	0.4404	0.7918	3.3614	0.2716
11	W, $^1\chi$	3.0019	0.4065	0.7773	3.0547	0.2589
12	Sz, $^1\chi$	2.9463	0.4283	0.7830	3.2474	0.2657

However, this model is to be discussed as the coefficients of both the terms involved *i.e.*, of W and Sz are quite smaller than their respective standard deviation and that such models are not allowed statistically. The data presented in Table 4.3.27 and 4.3.28 are consistent with our findings.

Table 4.3.27: Found and Estimated Antibacterial Activity of Mannich Bases against *B. subtilis* Using Best Model Containing Sz (Rooted graph)

Compound No.	*Found*	*Estimated*	*Residue*	*(Residue)^2*
1	18.05	15.68	2.37	5.6169
2	18.10	15.04	3.06	9.3636
3	13.31	12.79	0.52	0.2704
4	16.57	17.70	–1.13	1.2769
5	10.73	15.03	–4.30	18.49
7	9.49	9.67	–0.18	0.0324
8	9.47	9.79	–0.32	0.1024

Σ = 35.2353

From the results and discussion made above we conclude that the antibacterial activity of the Mannich bases used is not a global property and that it is influenced considerably by the substituent R.

Table 4.3.28: PE, LSE, LOF Values Calculated for the Derived Models for Modeling Antibacterial Activity of Mannich Bases against *B. subtilis* (Rooted graph)

Model	*Topological Index*	*PE*	*LSE*	*LOF*
1	W	0.1025	37.0729	454.14
2	Sz	0.0974	35.2352	431.63
3	$^1\chi$	0.1007	36.4390	446.37
4	J	0.2490	90.0347	1102.95
5	logRB	0.1017	36.7925	450.70
6	W, J	0.1024	37.0431	113.44
7	Sz, J	0.0972	35.1653	107.69
8	$^1\chi$, J	0.0980	35.4395	108.53
9	J, logRB	0.1017	36.7870	112.66
10	W, Sz	0.0940	33.9855	104.08
11	W, $^1\chi$	0.0997	36.0470	110.39
12	Sz, $^1\chi$	0.0975	34.7233	106.34

4.4. Modeling of Antibacterial Activity of Mannich Bases: 3,5-Dinitrobenzoyl-4-amino-benzamido-methyl Amines

The modeling a antibacterial activity of 3,5-dinitrobenzoyl-4-aminobenzamido-methyl amines against the three bacteria is carried out in similar manner *i.e.* by considering the entire molecular graphs as well as using rooted graphs.

4.4.1. Considering Entire Molecular Graphs of the Mannich Bases

The elemental analysis and adopted characterization are given in Tables 4.4.2 to 4.4.4.

The Mannich bases used are presented in Table 4.4.1. Their antibacterial activity against *E. coli* and *K. pneumonae* are given in Table 4.4.5. The calculated values of topological indices are presented in Table 4.4.6.

The correlation matrices for *E. coli* and *K. pneumonae* are recorded in Table 4.4.7. Proposed models are given in Table 4.4.8 and 4.4.11 respectively for *E. coli* and *K. pneumonae*.

Tables 4.4.7 and 4.4.8 show that no monoparametric models are possible for modeling antibacterial activity against *E. coli* and that a bi-parametric model contains Sz and $^1\chi$ gave the best model for modeling antibacterial activity against *E. coli*.

$$\text{Antibacterial activity against } E.\ coli = 63.1627 - 0.0038\ (\pm 0.0016)\ Sz - 4.4148\ (\pm 1.9390)\ {}^1\chi \quad (4.4.1)$$

$n = 6$, $Se = 2.3471$, $R = 0.8196$, $F = 3.069$, $Q = 0.3492$

The calculated values (Table 4.4.9) and the values of PE, LSE and LOF (Table 4.4.10) are in favour of this model.

Table 4.4.1: Name of the Mannich Bases along with their Molecular Structures

(1) 3,5-Dinitrobenzoyl-4-aminobenzamido methyl sulphadiazine

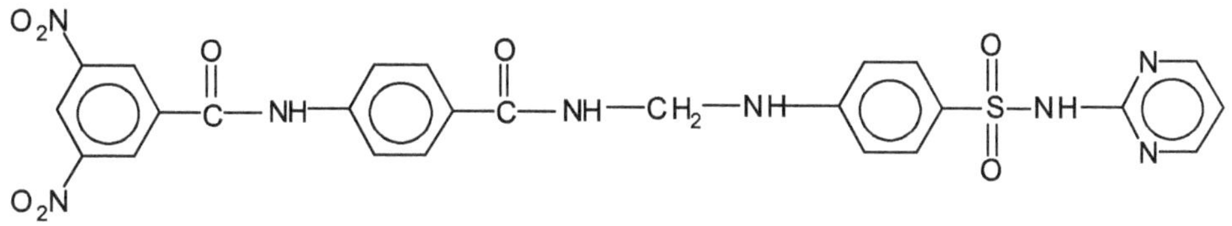

(2) 3,5-Dinitrobenzoyl-4-aminobenzamido methyl sulphamethoxazole

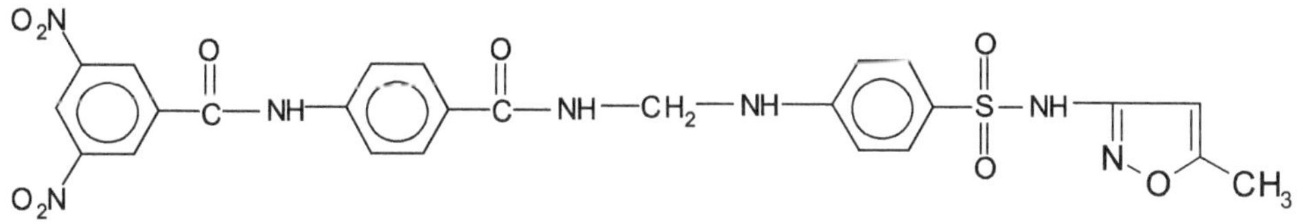

(3) 3,5-Dinitrobenzoyl-4-aminobenzamido methyl sulphaguanidine

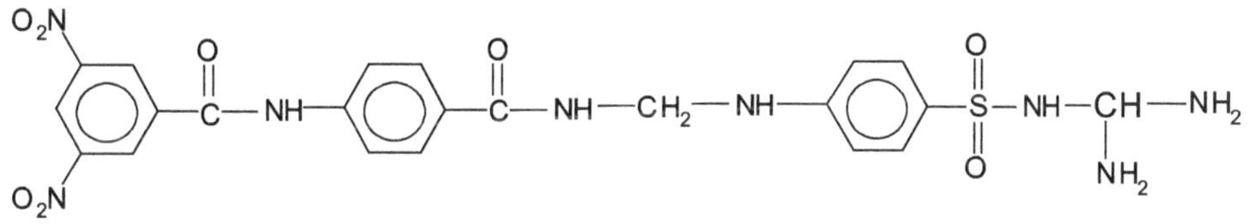

(4) 3,5-Dinitrobenzoyl-4-aminobenzamido methyl sulphadimidine

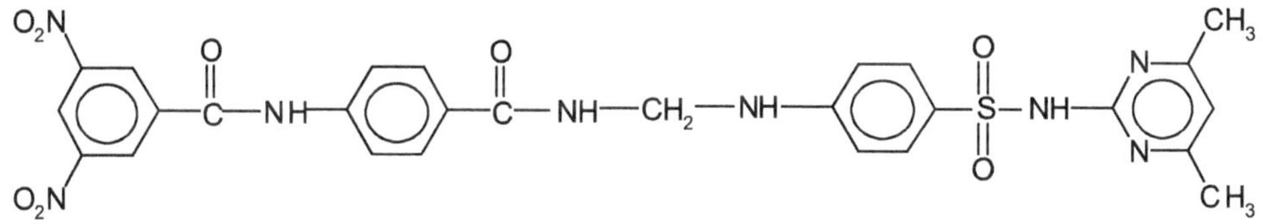

(5) 3,5-Dinitrobenzoyl-4-aminobenzamido methyl sulphamethiazole

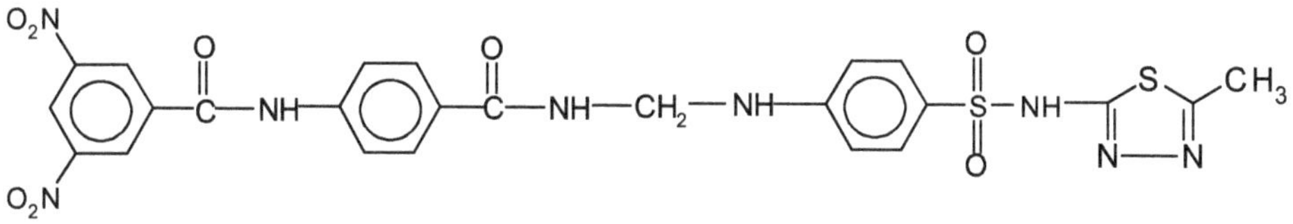

(6) 3,5-Dinitrobenzoyl-4-aminobenzamido methyl sulphanilamide

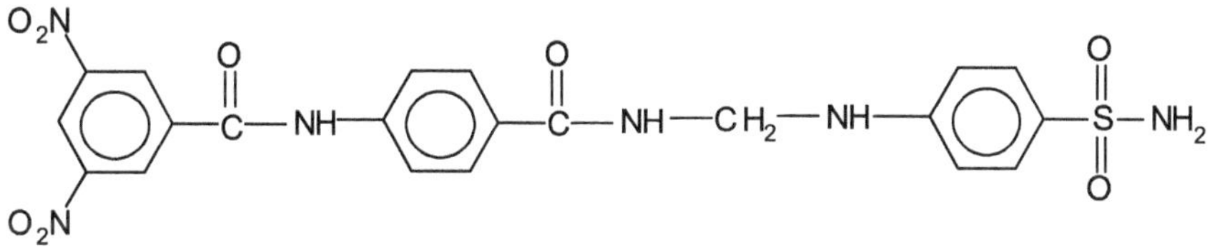

Contd...

Table 4.4.1–*Contd...*

(7) 3,5-Dinitrobenzoyl-4-aminobenzamido dimethyl amine

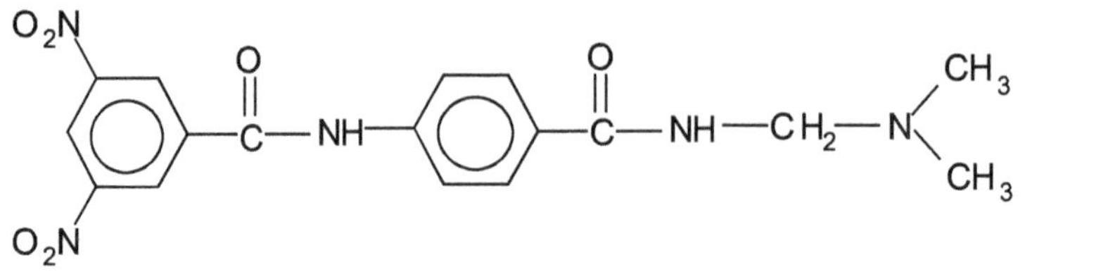

(8) 3,5-Dinitrobenzoyl-4-aminobenzamido diethyl amine

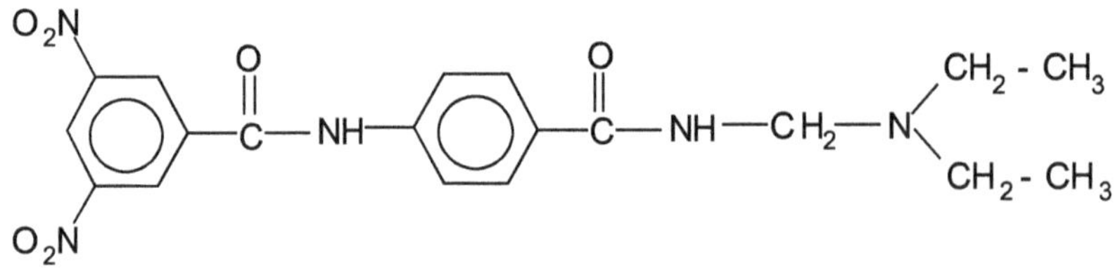

(9) 3,5-Dinitrobenzoyl-4-aminobenzamido diphenyl amine

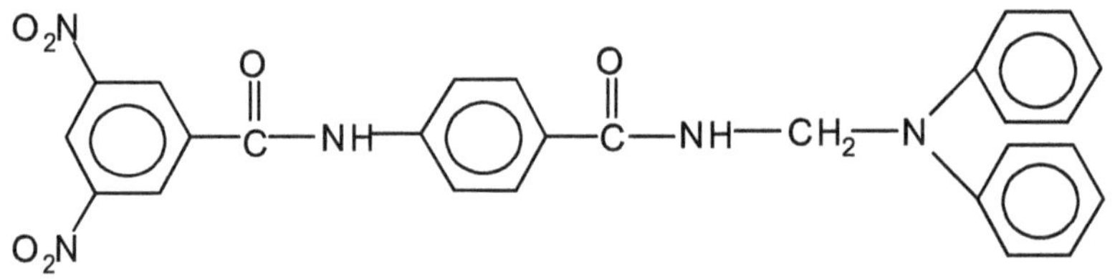

(10) 3,5-Dinitrobenzoyl-4-aminobenzamido diethanol amine

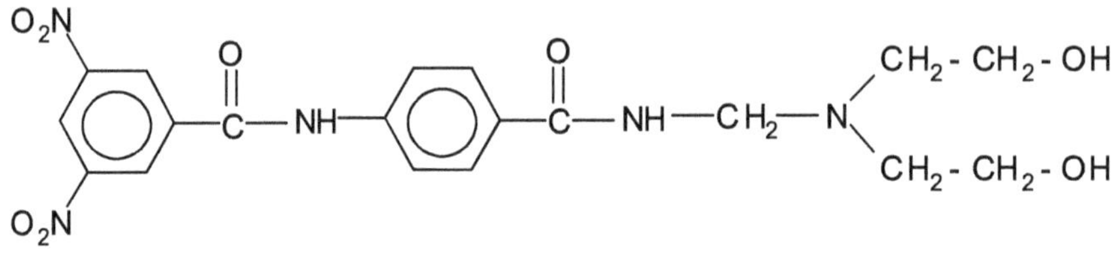

(11) 3,5-Dinitrobenzoyl-4-aminobenzamido morpholine

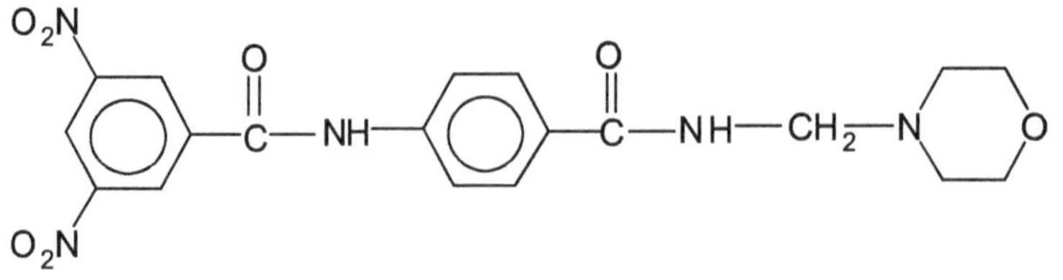

Contd...

Table 4.4.1–*Contd...*

(12) Bis-3,5-Dinitrobenzoyl-4-aminobenzamido methyl piperazine

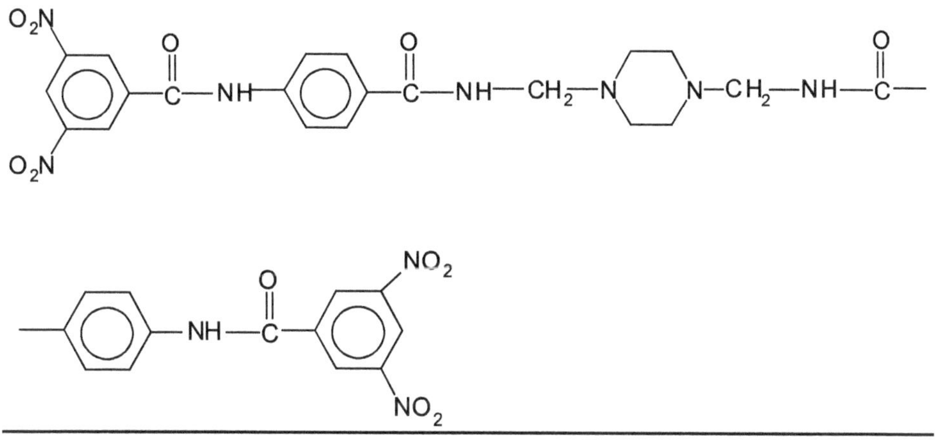

In case of *K. pneumonae* no model is found statistically significant (Table 4.4.11). However, the data did show that a biparametric model containing W and Sz indices are better for this purpose. The comparison of observed and calculated values for the activity (Table 4.4.12) as well as values of PE, LSE, LOF (Table 4.4.13) are in favour of this finding.

4.4.2. Results Obtained from Rooted Graphs

The rooted graphs, their topological indices and proposed matrices are given in Tables 4.4.14 to 16 respectively. The mono- and bi-parametric models for modeling anti-bacterial activity against *E. coli* as presented in Table 4.4.17 show that in no case statistically significant models are obtained. However, a model containing W and J is otherwise a good model.

$$\text{Antibacterial activity against } E.\ coli \text{ (Rooted)} = 2.9014 + 0.0043\ (\pm 0.0060)\ W + 6.8633\ (\pm 5.1819)\ J \qquad (4.4.2)$$

$n = 6$, $Se = 3.1272$, $R = 0.6459$, $F = 1.0738$, $Q = 0.2065$

The results recorded in Tables 4.4.18 and 4.4.19 are in favour of this findings.

Same is the case found for modeling antibacterial activity against *K. pneumonae* (Table 4.4.20), which again shows that the biparametric model containing Sz and $^1\chi$ is better.

$$\text{Antibacterial activity against } K.\ pneumonae \text{ (Rooted)} = 18.2671 - 0.00546\ (\pm 0.0037)\ Sz + 1.0047\ (\pm 1.3051)\ \chi^1 \qquad (4.4.3)$$

$n = 11$, $Se = 6.9572$, $R = 0.5634$, $F = 1.8597$, $Q = 0.0809$

Table 4.4.2: Characterization Data of 3,5-Dinitrobenzoyl-4-aminobenzamido-methyl Amines

Sl.No.	*Compound*	*Mol. Formula*	*m.p. (°C)*	*Elemental Analysis Found (Calcd.) %*		
				C	*H*	*N*
1.	3,5-Dinitrobenzoyl-4-aminobenzamido-methyl sulphadiazine	$C_{25}H_{20}N_8O_8S$	128-130	50.30 (50.67	2.92 3.37	18.59 18.91)
2.	3,5-Dinitrobenzoyl-4-aminobenzamidomethyl-sulphamethoxazole	$C_{25}H_{21}N_7O_9S$	137	50.90 (50.42	3.80 3.52	16.70 16.47)
3.	3,5-Dinitrobenzoyl-4-aminobenzamidomethyl-sulphaguanidine	$C_{22}H_{20}N_8O_8S$	120	47.83 (47.48	3.70 3.59	20.40 20.14)
4.	3,5-Dinitrobenzoyl-4-aminobenzamidomethyl-sulphadimidine	$C_{27}H_{24}N_8O_8S$	95-97	52.01 (52.25	3.52 3.87	17.79 18.06)
5.	3,5-Dinitrobenzoyl-4-aminobenzamidomethyl-sulphamethiazole	$C_{24}H_{20}N_8O_8S_2$	190	47.40 (47.05	3.61 3.26	18.65 18.30)
6.	3,5-Dinitrobenzoyl-4-aminobenzamidomethyl-sulphanilamide	$C\text{-}_{21}H_{18}N_6O_8S$	98-100	48.68 (49.02	3.04 3.50	15.89 16.34)
7.	3,5-Dinitrobenzoyl-4-aminobenzamidomethyl-dimethylamine	$C\text{-}_{17}H_{17}N_5O_6$	100-102	52.36 (52.71	3.96 4.39	17.72 18.08)
8.	3,5-Dinitrobenzoyl-4-aminobenzamidomethyl-diethylamine	$C\text{-}_{19}H_{21}N_5O_6$	65	54.58 (54.93	4.71 5.06	17.01 16.86)
9.	3,5-Dinitrobenzoyl-4-aminobenzamidomethyl-diphenylamine	$C\text{-}_{27}H_{21}N_5O_6$	89-90	62.98 (63.40	446 4.10	14.00 13.69)
10.	3,5-Dinitrobenzoyl-4-aminobenzamidomethyl-diethanolamine	$C\text{-}_{19}H_{21}N_5O_8$	110-112	50.68 (51.00	4.27 4.69	15.19 15.65)
11.	3,5-Dinitrobenzoyl-4-aminobenzamidomethyl-morpholine	$C\text{-}_{19}H_{19}N_5O_7$	85	53.48 (53.14	4.90 4.42	16.81 16.31)
12.	3,5-Dinitrobenzoyl-4-aminobenzamidomethyl-piperazine	$C\text{-}_{34}H_{30}N_{10}O_{12}$	132-133	52.60 (52.98	3.40 3.89	17.65 18.18)

Table 4.4.3: Ir Frequency Bands of 3,5-dinitrobenzoyl-4-aminobenzamido Methyl Amines

I	*II*	*III*	*IV*	*V*	*VI*	*VII*	*VIII*	*IX*	*X*	*XI*	*XII*
3450(s)	3400(m)	3450(m)	3475(s)	3350(m)	3440(w)	3499(s)	3420(m)	3450(s)	3350(s)	3401(m)	3250(m)
3360(s)	3190(m)	3340(s)	3380(s)	3100(m)	3300	3400(s)	3100(m)	3100(s)	3170(w)	3325(s)	3195(sh)
3100(s)	3100(s)	3150(m)	3320(sh)	3050	3100(w)	3100(m)	2995	3000(m)	1660(m)	3100(m)	3100(m)
3050(s)	3040(m)	3025(m)	3170(w)	2980	2900(w)	2860(w)	2940	2940(s)	1601(s)	3000(w)	3000(m)
2940(s)	2960(m)	2900(w)	3100(s)	2900(w)	1680(m)	2770(w)	2840(w)	2880(s)	1535(s)	2902(w)	2950
2870(s)	2940(m)	2799(w)	3025(w)	2800(w)	1655(s)	2700	2780(w)	2725	1450(m)	2850(w)	2900(w)
2800(s)	2860(s)	1675(m)	2840(w)	1660(m)	1599(s)	1680(m)	1680(s)	1650(s)	1380(m)	1665(m)	2750
2730(s)	2800(m)	1615(m)	2780	1600(s)	1535(m)	1619(m)	1660(sh)	1681(sh)	1348(s)	1605(s)	1650(m)
1680(m)	1680(m)	1575(m)	1675(m)	1582(sh)	1460(m)	1595(s)	1630(m)	1601(s)	1320(w)	1573(sh)	1600(s)
1650(s)	1598(s)	1530(m)	1630(m)	1530(m)	1410(s)	1535(m)	1600(s)	1535(s)	1250(m)	1530(m)	1535(s)
1595(s)	1538(s)	1455(w)	1598(s)	1450(s)	1345(s)	1500	1538(s)	1455(s)	1175(m)	1490(sh)	1455(s)
1580(sh)	1510(sh)	1400(s)	1450(m)	1410(s)	1320(s)	1470(s)	1470(w)	1430(w)	1070(s)	1455(m)	1382(m)
1551(s)	1464(s)	1345(s)	1435(m)	1345(s)	1260(m)	1400(s)	1455(m)	1403(s)	1030(sh)	1405(w)	1345(s)
1490(s)	1400(s)	1300(w)	1385(m)	1325(s)	1240(m)	1342(s)	1410(m)	1375(s)	920(m)	1380(w)	1312(m)
1440(s)	1340(s)	1260(w)	1343(s)	1290(s)	1145(s)	1327(w)	1380(m)	1345(s)	785(m)	1345(s)	1261(m)
1410(s)	1320(s)	1230(s)	1300(m)	1275(m)	1090(m)	1300(w)	1345(s)	1320(m)	720(s)	1310(m)	1232(m)
1345(s)	1260(m)	1172(s)	1265(m)	1250(s)	1015(m)	1265(s)	1320(m)	1260(m)	670(w)	1260(w)	1170(s)
1325(s)	1242(sh)	1080(s)	1189(s)	1190(s)	955(w)	1190(s)	1260(m)	1240(m)		1240(w)	1085(m)
1260(s)	1158(s)	1010(w)	1150(s)	1139(s)	910(m)	1158(s)	1179(s)	1175(s)		1170(s)	1070(m)
1155(s)	1140(sh)	920(s)	1080(s)	1090(s)	820(s)	1132(sh)	1120(w)	1190(sh)		1072(m)	1010(w)
1092(s)	1090(s)	820(s)	1032(m)	1030(m)	765(s)	1090(s)	1075(m)	1105(s)		1010(w)	982(w)
998(m)	1030(m)	760(w)	1010(m)	1000(m)	718(s)	1035(m)	1010(w)	1045(s)	920(s)	950(w)	

Contd...

Table 4.4.3–*Contd...*

I	*II*	*III*	*IV*	*V*	*VI*	*VII*	*VIII*	*IX*	*X*	*XI*	*XII*
940(s)	1000(m)	720(s)	973(m)	917(s)	670(w)	1005(m)	918(m)	920(s)		800(m)	915(s)
840(s)	959(m)	682(s)	920(s)	830(s)		920(m)	855(m)	900(s)		770(s)	855(m)
825(s)	920(s)	653(w)	855(m)	770(m)		885(m)	770(s)	871(s)		750(m)	835(m)
799(s)	870(m)		830(m)	700(s)		830(s)	728(s)	850(sh)		720(s)	780(m)
760(w)	821(s)		790(s)	650(s)		789(s)	710(sh)	815(w)		690(s)	760(sh)
720(s)	800(w)		760(w)			720(s)	668(w)	790(m)		670(sh)	715(s)
680(s)	771(m)		720(s)			685(s)		770(m)			690(w)
720(s)		670(s)					725(s)				
680(s)							710(s)				
690(w)											
667(m)											

(m) = medium, (s) = strong, (w) = weak, (sh) = shoulder.

The results obtained recorded in Table 4.4.21 and 4.4.22 are in favour of this finding.

The results once again show that antibacterial activity is influenced by the effect due to substutient R.

Table 4.4.4: ^{1}H NMR Spectral Data of 3,5-dinitrobenzoyl-4-aminobenzene Amidomethyl Amines

Compd. No.	*δ values in ppm*					
	CH_2 (d)	*NH (s)*	*Various (m) Ring Protons*	*CONH of Ring I (s)*	*CONH of Ring II (t)*	*SO_2NH (s)*
I	2.8	6.1	6.6 – 8.9	7.7	8.3	11.0
II	2.6	6.1	6.6 – 8.8	7.7	8.0	11.08
III	2.55	6.09	6.55 – 8.9	7.85	8.0	11.1
IV	2.4	6.0	6.6 – 8.9	7.85	7.93	11.12
V	2.49	6.1	6.9 – 9.0	7.8	8.28	11.2
VI	2.55	6.1	6.78 – 9.1	7.5	8.37	11.08
VII	2.4	–	6.7 – 9.0	7.85	7.9	–
VIII	2.5	–	6.7 – 9.1	7.91	8.3	–
IX	2.55	–	6.5 – 9.2	7.73	8.28	–
X	2.5	–	6.62 – 9.2	7.9	8.3	–
XI	2.5	–	6.6 – 9.0	7.9	8.29	–
XII	2.5	–	6.55 – 9.2	7.58	8.0	–

(d) = doublet; (s) = singlet; (m) = multiplet; (t) = triplet.

Table 4.4.5: Antibacterial Activity of Mannich Bases

Compound No.	*Zone of Inhibition in mm*				*Average*
	Concentration in µg/ml				
	10	*20*	*40*	*80*	
(A) Against *E. coli*					
1	14.80	17.66	21.76	24.20	19.60
2	15.93	18.80	20.06	21.63	19.10
5	14.10	16.36	18.10	19.60	17.04
6	19.13	21.06	18.90	19.73	19.70
7	14.76	16.23	14.76	20.30	16.51
9	6.10	10.20	13.66	15.43	11.35
(B) Against *K. pneumonae*					
1	27.26	27.30	17.96	22.10	23.75
2	16.43	23.60	27.30	25.06	23.10

Contd...

Table 4.4.5–*Contd...*

Compound No.	*Zone of Inhibition in mm*				*Average*
	Concentration in μg/ml				
	10	*20*	*40*	*80*	
3	27.83	28.40	27.90	27.90	28.00
4	6.00	23.00	19.53	23.56	18.02
6	9.10	9.73	9.43	9.20	9.36
7	23.66	29.66	25.83	26.70	26.45
8	19.16	7.03	7.33	29.76	15.82
9	27.16	27.00	28.53	26.40	27.27
10	26.40	29.96	29.13	27.96	28.36
11	19.56	26.00	6.10	7.03	14.67
12	6.00	6.13	8.96	9.46	7.64

Table 4.4.6: Distance Based Topological Indices Calculated for Mannich Bases

Compound No.	*W*	*Sz*	*$^1\chi$*	*J*	*logRB*
1	8158	11665	20.0128	1.0980	1696.3320
2	8157	11428	19.9067	1.0987	1695.9270
3	6566	9236	18.3511	1.3257	1415.2010
4	9268	13281	20.8006	1.1025	1894.9760
5	8157	11428	19.9067	1.0987	1695.9270
6	5173	7357	16.9346	1.3358	1159.6390
7	2357	3332	13.1676	1.8003	606.3539
8	2915	4040	14.2436	1.7785	725.7615
9	5527	7882	18.3126	1.2188	1279.9350
10	3543	4818	15.2436	1.7650	856.9139
11	3218	4670	14.8294	1.3967	787.4462
12	16563	26407	26.4087	0.8699	2932.4850

Table 4.4.7: Correlation Matrix for Modeling Antibacterial Activity of Mannich Bases

	Activity	*W*	*Sz*	*$^1\chi$*	*J*	*logRB*
(A) For *E. coli*						
Activity	1.0000					
W	0.32426	1.0000				
Sz	0.32318	0.99961	1.0000			
$^1\chi$	0.16435	0.97727	0.97938	1.0000		
J	–0.14090	–0.95311	–0.95596	–0.99295	1.0000	
logRB	0.27133	0.99754	0.99785	0.98969	–0.97102	1.0000

Contd...

Table 4.4.7–*Contd...*

	Activity	W	Sz	$^1\chi$	J	logRB
(B) For *K. pneumonae*						
Activity	1.0000					
W	–0.4224	1.0000				
Sz	–0.4535	0.9971	1.0000			
$^1\chi$	–0.3559	0.9859	0.9742	1.0000		
J	0.3385	–0.8525	–0.8280	–0.9078	1.0000	
logRB	–0.3840	0.9959	0.9869	0.9958	–0.8844	1.0000

Table 4.4.8: Regression Analysis and Quality of Correlations for Modeling Antibacterial Activity of Mannich Bases against *E. coli*

Model	Topological Index	Se	R^2_A	R	F	Q
1	W	3.3559	–	0.3243	0.470	0.0966
2	Sz	3.3572	–	0.3232	0.467	0.0962
3	$^1\chi$	3.4994	–	0.1644	0.111	0.0470
4	J	3.5122	–	–0.1409	0.081	0.0401
5	logRB	3.4145	–	0.2713	0.381	0.0794
6	W, J	3.1362	0.0231	0.6433	1.059	0.2051
7	Sz, J	3.0865	0.0539	0.6575	1.142	0.2130
8	$^1\chi$, J	3.9666	–0.5627	0.2497	0.100	0.0629
9	J, logRB	3.3365	–0.1057	0.5802	0.761	0.1739
10	W, Sz	3.8726	–0.4895	0.3260	0.178	0.0842
11	W, $^1\chi$	2.5160	0.3713	0.7892	2.476	0.3137
12	Sz, $^1\chi$	2.3471	0.4529	0.8196	3.069	0.3492

Table 4.4.9: Found and Estimated Antibacterial Activity of Mannich Bases against *E. coli* Using Best Model Containing Sz, $^1\chi$

Compound No.	Observed Activity	Estimated Activity	Residue	$(Residue)^2$
1	19.60	19.24	0.36	0.1296
2	19.10	18.80	0.30	0.0900
5	17.04	18.80	–1.76	3.0976
6	19.70	16.42	3.28	10.7584
7	16.51	17.20	–0.69	0.4761
9	11.35	12.33	–0.98	0.9604

$\Sigma = 15.5263$

Table 4.4.10: PE, LSE, LOF Values Calculated for the Derived Models for Modeling Antibacterial Activity of Mannich Bases against *E. coli*

Model	*Topological Index*	*PE*	*LSE*	*LOF*
1	W	0.2434	45.0493	405.4441
2	Sz	0.2436	45.0844	405.7596
3	$^1\chi$	0.2647	48.9827	440.8443
4	J	0.2667	49.3431	444.0879
5	logRB	0.2520	46.6362	419.7258
6	W, J	0.1595	29.5073	66.3914
7	Sz, J	0.1544	28.5787	64.3020
8	$^1\chi$, J	0.2551	47.2026	106.2058
9	J, logRB	0.1804	33.3975	75.1444
10	W, Sz	0.2431	44.9915	101.2308
11	W, $^1\chi$	0.1026	18.9911	42.7299
12	Sz, $^1\chi$	0.0893	15.5263	34.9341

Table 4.4.11: Regression Analysis and Quality of Correlations for Modeling Antibacterial Activity of Mannich Bases against *K. pneumonae*

Model	*Topological Index*	*Se*	R^2_A	*R*	*F*	*Q*
1	W	7.1959	–	–0.4224	1.9547	0.0587
2	Sz	7.07562	–	–0.4535	2.3303	0.0641
3	$^1\chi$	7.4192	–	–0.3559	1.3053	0.0479
4	J	7.4703	–	0.3385	1.1648	0.0453
5	logRB	7.3302	–	–0.38404	1.5156	0.0523
6	W, J	7.6245	–0.0248	0.4244	0.8789	0.0556
7	Sz, J	7.4842	0.0125	0.4583	1.0636	0.0612
8	$^1\chi$, J	7.8632	–0.0899	0.3578	0.5873	0.0455
9	J, logRB	7.7749	–0.0656	0.3840	0.6920	0.0494
10	W, Sz	6.7231	0.2032	0.6021	2.2749	0.0896
11	W, $^1\chi$	6.9978	0.1367	0.5562	1.7920	0.0795
12	Sz, $^1\chi$	6.7859	0.1882	0.5921	2.1594	0.0872

Table 4.4.12: Found and estimated antibacterial activity of Mannich bases against *K. pneumonae* using best model having W and Sz indices

Compound No.	Found	Estimated	Residue	(Residue)^2
1	23.75	22.54	1.21	1.4641
2	23.10	24.06	–0.96	0.9216
3	28.00	22.88	5.12	26.2144
4	18.02	22.79	–4.77	22.7530
6	9.36	21.58	–12.22	149.3280
7	26.45	20.43	6.02	36.2400
8	15.82	21.23	–5.41	29.2680
9	27.27	21.61	5.66	32.0355
10	28.36	22.27	6.09	37.0880
11	14.67	20.07	–5.40	29.1600
12	7.64	8.24	–0.60	0.3600

Σ = 361.6030

Table 4.4.13: PE, LSE, LOF Values Calculated for the Derived Models for Modeling Antibacterial Activity of Mannich Bases against *K. pneumonae*

Model	Topological Index	PE	LSE	LOF
1	W	0.1651	466.0367	14122.32
2	Sz	0.1596	450.5797	13651.50
3	$^1\chi$	0.1755	495.4052	15012.12
4	J	0.1779	502.2507	15212.12
5	logRB	0.1713	483.5940	14654.54
6	W, J	0.1648	465.0700	3515.26
7	Sz, J	0.1587	448.1094	3386.99
8	$^1\chi$, J	0.1752	494.6368	3738.47
9	J, logRB	0.1713	483.5907	3655.32
10	W, Sz	0.1281	361.6030	2733.18
11	W, $^1\chi$	0.1388	391.7525	2961.07
12	Sz, $^1\chi$	0.1305	368.3859	2784.58

Table 4.4.14: All H Suppressed Rooted Graphs of Mannich Bases

General Structure: 3,5-Dinitrobenzoyl-4-aminobenzamido methyl amines

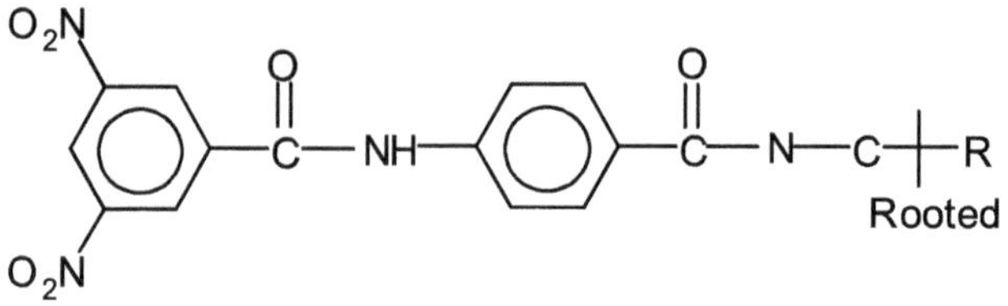

O_2N O_2N O O C—NH— C—N—C—R Rooted

R =

1\.

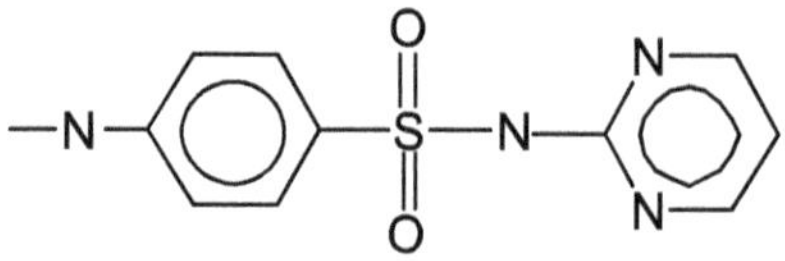

2\.

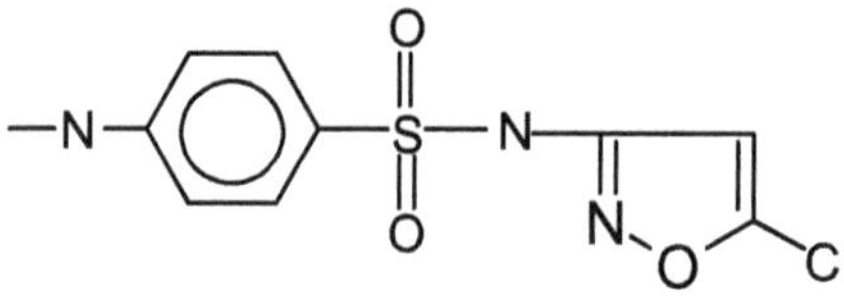

3\.

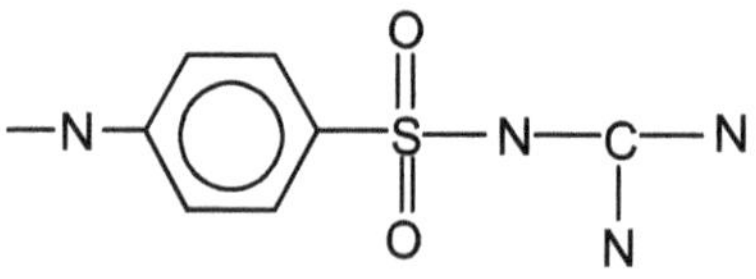

4\.

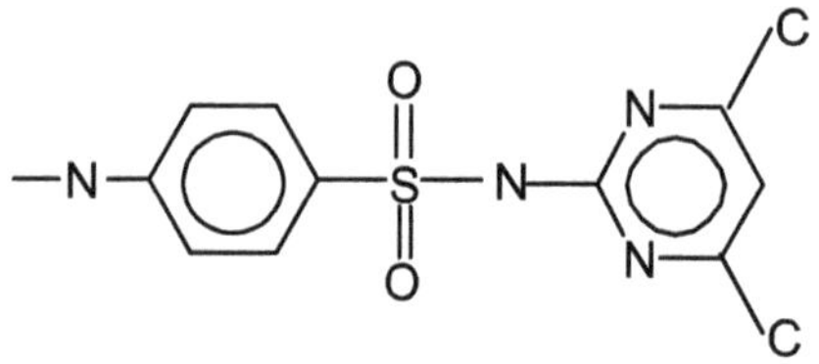

5\.

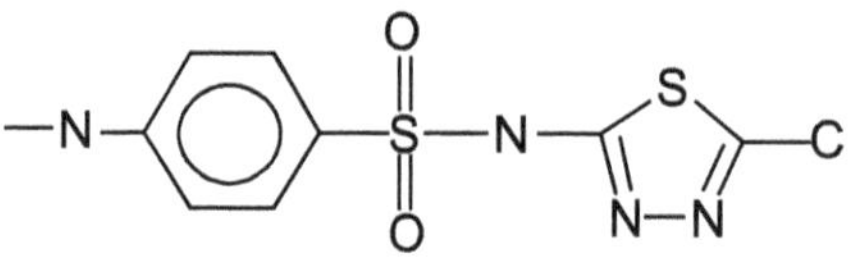

Contd...

Table 4.4.14–*Contd...*

6.

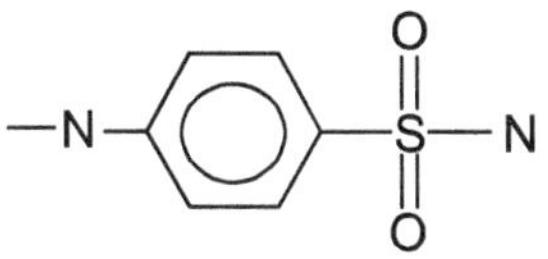

7.

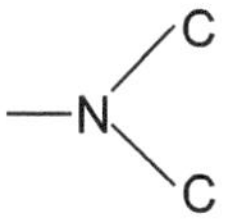

8.

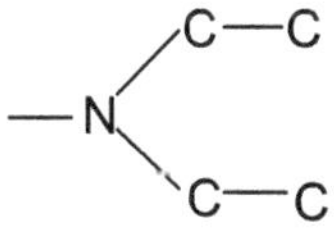

9.

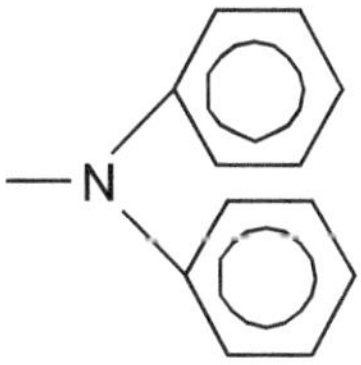

10.

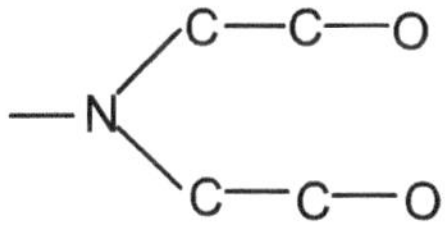

11.

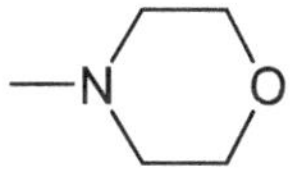

12.

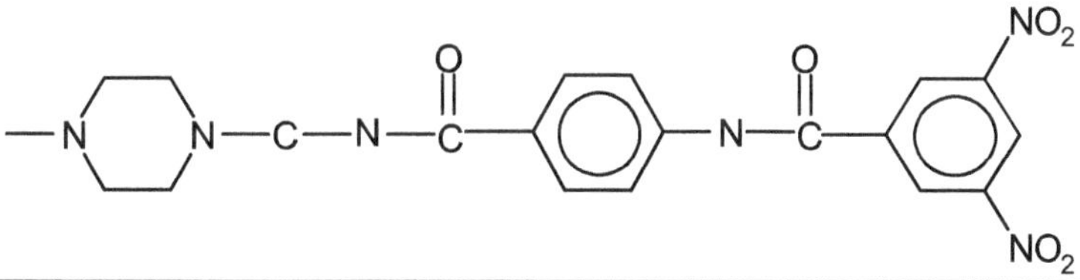

Table 4.4.15: Distance Based Topological Indices Calculated for Mannich Bases (Rooted graph)

Compound No.	*W*	*Sz*	$^1\chi$	*J*	*logRB*
1	536	818	8.0773	1.8372	162.0572
2	535	731	7.9712	1.8479	161.6517
3	307	427	6.4155	2.4613	96.2437
4	722	1092	8.8650	1.8868	215.2262
5	535	731	7.9712	1.8479	161.6517
6	152	236	4.9990	2.3936	48.2757
7	4	4	1.4142	1.6330	0.6931
8	20	20	2.4142	2.1906	5.6630
9	264	444	6.4495	1.6872	81.3185
10	56	56	3.4142	2.4478	17.0297
11	27	54	3.0000	2.0000	7.4547
12	3218	4670	14.8294	1.3967	787.4468

Table 4.4.16: Correlation Matrix for the Calculation of Antibacterial Activity of Mannich Bases (Rooted graph)

	Activity	*W*	*Sz*	$^1\chi$	*J*	*logRB*
(A) For *E. coli*						
Activity	1.0000					
W	0.2765	1.0000				
Sz	0.2283	0.9918	1.0000			
$^1\chi$	0.1550	0.9483	0.9640	1.0000		
J	0.5650	–0.0635	–0.0704	0.0909	1.0000	
logRB	0.2753	0.9998	0.9926	0.9528	–0.0526	1.0000
(B) For *K. pneumonae*						
Activity	1.0000					
W	–0.5144	1.0000				
Sz	–0.5165	0.9997	1.0000			
$^1\chi$	–0.3636	0.8936	0.8967	1.0000		
J	0.1667	–0.5884	–0.5960	–0.4998	1.0000	
logRB	–0.4982	0.9979	0.9980	0.9187	–0.5900	1.0000

Table 4.4.17: Regression Analysis and Quality of Correlation for Modeling Antibacterial Activity of Mannich Bases against *E. coli* (Rooted graph)

Model	*Topological Index*	*Se*	R^2_A	*R*	*F*	*Q*
1	W	3.4093	–	0.2765	0.3310	0.0811
2	Sz	3.4539	–	0.2283	0.2200	0.0661
3	$^1\chi$	3.5047	–	0.1550	0.0985	0.0442
4	J	2.9270	–	0.5650	1.8759	0.1930
5	logRB	3.4105	–	0.2753	0.3279	0.0807
6	W, J	3.1272	0.0287	0.6459	1.0738	0.2065
7	Sz, J	3.1954	–0.0141	0.6257	0.9652	0.1958
8	$^1\chi$, J	3.3528	–0.1165	0.5745	0.7391	0.1713
9	J, logRB	3.13973	0.0209	0.6420	1.0534	0.2044
10	W, Sz	3.6500	–0.3232	0.4539	0.3893	0.1243
11	W, $^1\chi$	3.6862	–0.3495	0.4362	0.3524	0.1183
12	Sz, $^1\chi$	3.8599	–0.4797	0.3349	0.1895	0.0867

Table 4.4.18: Found and Estimated Antibacterial Activity of Mannich Bases against *E. coli* Using Best Model Containing W, J (Rooted graph)

Compound No.	Found	Estimated	Residue	$(Residue)^2$
1	19.60	17.81	1.79	3.2041
2	19.10	17.87	1.23	1.5129
5	17.04	17.87	–0.83	0.6889
6	19.70	19.97	–0.27	0.0729
7	16.51	14.13	2.38	5.6644
9	11.35	15.61	–4.26	18.1476

$\Sigma = 29.3387$

Table 4.4.19: PE, LSE, LOF Values Calculated for the Derived Models for Modeling Antibacterial Activity of Mannich Bases against *E. coli* (Rooted graph)

Model	Topological Index	PE	LSE	LOF
1	W	0.2513	46.4944	418.44
2	Sz	0.2579	47.7175	429.45
3	$^1\chi$	0.2655	49.1332	442.19
4	J	0.1852	34.2704	308.43
5	logRB	0.2514	46.5279	418.75
6	W, J	0.1585	29.3387	66.01
7	Sz, J	0.1655	30.6320	68.92
8	$^1\chi$, J	0.1823	33.7244	75.87
9	J, logRB	0.1599	29.5738	66.54
10	W, Sz	0.2160	39.9629	89.91
11	W, $^1\chi$	0.2203	40.7641	91.72
12	Sz, $^1\chi$	0.2415	44.6961	100.56

Table 4.4.20: Regression Analysis and Quality of Correlations for Modeling Antibacterial Activity of Mannich Bases against *K. pneumonae* (Rooted graph)

Model	Topological Index	Se	R^2_A	R	F	Q
1	W	6.8079	–	–0.5144	3.2392	0.0755
2	Sz	6.7979	–	–0.5165	3.2751	0.0759
3	$^1\chi$	7.3956	–	–0.3636	1.3713	0.0491
4	J	7.8279	–	0.1667	0.2572	0.0213
5	logRB	6.8835	–	–0.4982	2.9716	0.0723
6	W, J	7.0805	0.1162	0.5412	1.6574	0.0764
7	Sz, J	7.0566	0.1221	0.5456	1.6957	0.0773

Contd...

Table 4.4.20–*Contd...*

Model	Topological Index	Se	R^2_A	R	F	Q
8	$^1\chi$, J	7.8428	–0.0843	0.3640	0.6110	0.0464
9	J, logRB	7.1794	0.0913	0.5225	1.5026	0.0727
10	W, Sz	7.1781	0.09167	0.5228	1.5046	0.0728
11	W, $^1\chi$	6.9923	0.1381	0.5604	1.8011	0.0801
12	Sz, $^1\chi$	6.9572	0.1467	0.5634	1.8597	0.0809

Table 4.4.21: Found and Estimated Antibacterial Activity of Mannich Bases against *K. pneumonae* Using Best Model Containing W, $^1\chi$ (Rooted graph)

Compound No.	Found	Estimated	Residue	$(Residue)^2$
1	23.75	21.92	1.83	3.3489
2	23.10	22.28	0.82	0.6724
3	28.00	22.38	5.62	31.5844
4	18.02	21.20	–3.18	10.1124
6	9.36	21.97	–12.61	159.0121
7	26.45	19.66	6.79	46.1041
8	15.82	20.57	–4.75	22.5625
9	27.27	22.32	4.95	24.5025
10	28.36	21.39	6.97	48.5809
11	14.67	20.98	–6.31	39.8161
12	7.64	7.66	–0.02	0.0004

$\Sigma = 387.22$

Table 4.4.22: PE, LSE, LOF Values Calculated for the Derived Models for Modeling Antibacterial Activity of Mannich Bases Against *K. pneumonae* (Rooted graph)

Model	Topological Index	PE	LSE	LOF
1	W	0.1478	417.1273	12640.22
2	Sz	0.1473	415.9077	12603.03
3	$^1\chi$	0.1744	492.2535	14916.66
4	J	0.1954	551.4926	16712.12
5	logRB	0.1511	426.4507	12922.72
6	W, J	0.1421	401.0684	3033.73
7	Sz, J	0.1411	398.3706	3013.38
8	$^1\chi$, J	0.1743	492.0826	3722.24
9	J, logRB	0.1461	412.3571	3119.19
10	W, Sz	0.1460	412.2038	3118.03
11	W, $^1\chi$	0.1368	391.1393	2958.69
12	Sz, $^1\chi$	0.1372	387.2222	2929.06

4.5. QSAR Study on the Antibacterial Activity of Newly Synthesized Mannich Bases Derived from 3,5-dinitrobenzoyl-4-aminobenzaqmido-methyl Amines: Considering only Carbon-Hydrogen Suppressed Graph

4.5.1. Introduction

Mannich base is the result of the condensation of a compound capable of supplying one or more active hydrogen atoms with aldehyde and ammonia or primary and secondary amines. Several biological active and medicinally useful Mannich bases have been critically reviewed by Tramontini, Angiolini and Ghedini[1]. Because of the biological significance and tremendous use of sulfonamides in pharmaceutical and medicinal chemistry several Mannich bases have been synthesised from sulfonamides using Mannich reaction[2]. Most of Mannich bases are found more active and less toxic than the parent compounds. This is found to be the case with Mannich bases derived from sulfonamides. The versatile utility of the Mannich bases in polymers, dispersants in the lubricating oil and in pharmaceutical and medicinal chemistry promoted us to synthesis and evaluate several Mannich bases from sulfonamides[3–9], flubendazole[10,11], mebenzazole[12,13], albendazole[14–16] etc. and screened them for their antimicrobial activities. However, a detailed structure-activity relationship (SAR) has not been attempted so far. Although a qualitative treatment on SAR has been given in our earlier communications[3–16]. This has promoted us to undertake the present investigation, in that we have modeled antibacterial activities of Mannich bases synthesized from 3,5-dinitrobenzoyl-4-aminobenzaqmido-methyl amines (Figure 4.5.1) against *E. coli* and *K. pneumonae* using distance based topological indices.

The results as discussed below indicate that we can use distance-based topological indices successfully for modeling, monitoring, and estimating antibacterial activity of Mannich bases under present investigation.

4.5.2. Results and Discussion

Before discussing our results it is worthy to mention that QSAR[22–27] is a major factor in contemporary drug design and that topological method gained maximum popularity in QSAR study in late 70's and early 80's with successful application in many fitting/predictive problems. Since then, the use of topological indices in QSAR has become a growing importance. The main reason for this is that topological indices report translations of molecular structures into characteristic structural descriptors expressed as numerical indices which may then be used in QSAR studies. Out of the several such indices used, those used in the present investigation are:

Wiener (W)- (Ref.17), first order molecular connectivity (${}^1\chi$) (Ref.18), Balaban (J)- (Ref.19), and Szeged (Sz)- (Ref.20,21) index and these indices were found more useful in QSAR/QSPR/QSTR studies.

A perusal of Table 4.5.1 shows that out of 12 Mannich bases only **1,2,5,6,7** and **9** are found active against *E. coli* and that the Mannich base 6 is most active against *E. coli*. The relative potential of the Mannich bases against *E. coli* is found as below:

I (1 – 6)

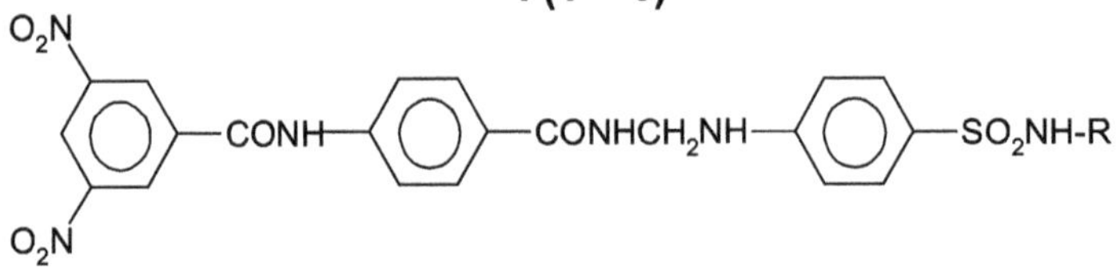

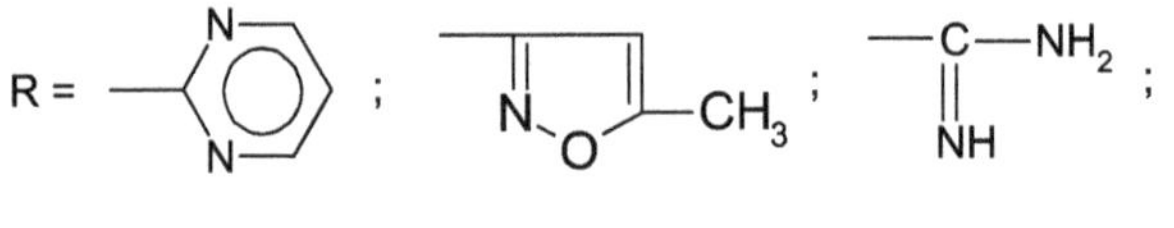

(1) (2) (3)

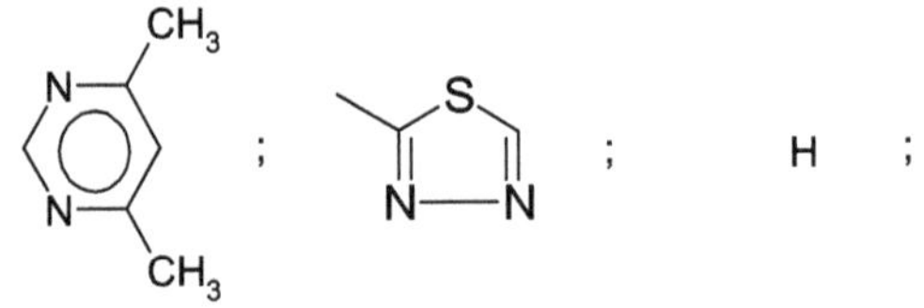

(4) (5) (6)

II (7 – 10)

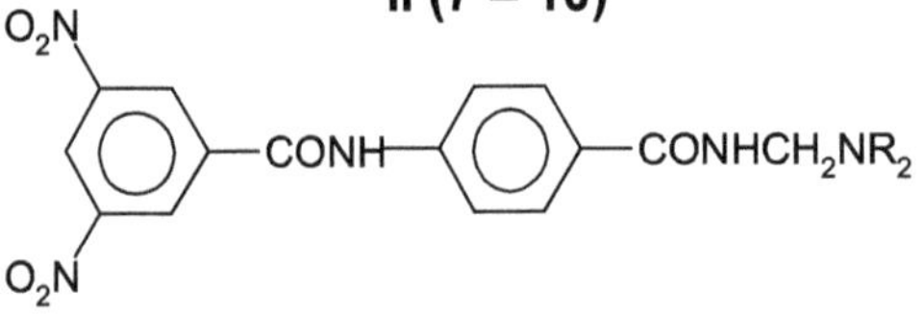

R = $-CH_3$; $-C_2H_5$; $-C_6H_5$; $-C_2H_4OH$

(7) (8) (9) (10)

III (11 – 12)

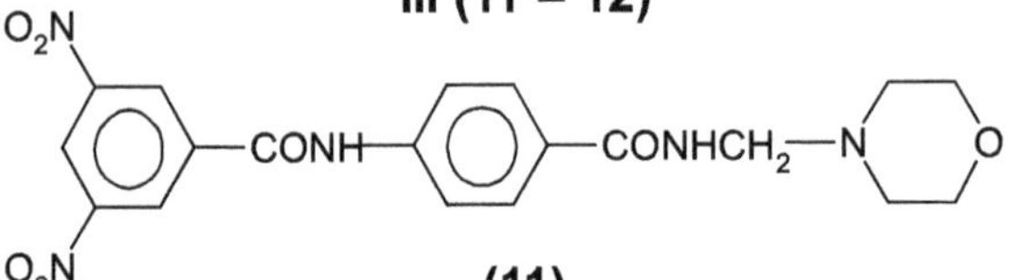

(11)

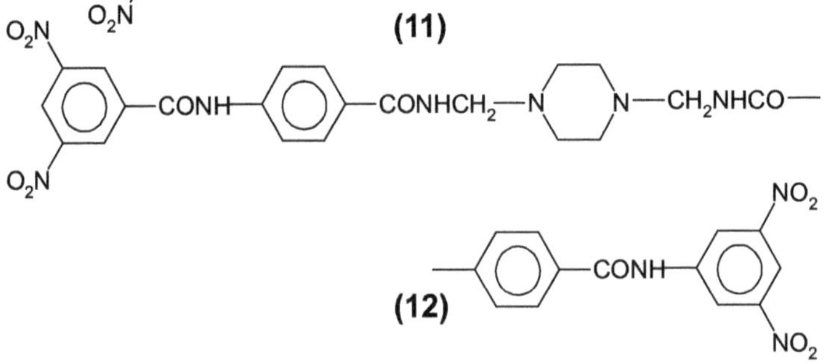

(12)

Figure 4.5.1: Structural Details of Mannich Bases Synthesized by us and Used in the Present Investigation.

Table 4.5.1: Mannich Bases, their Antibacterial Activities against *E. coli* and *K. pneumonae* and Indicator Parameters

Comp No.	*E. coli*					*K. pneumonae*					IP_1	IP_2
	Zone of Inhibition in mm.					*Zone of Inhibition in mm.*						
	Concentration in µg/ml					*Concentration in µg/ml*						
	10	*20*	*40*	*80*	*Avg*	*10*	*20*	*40*	*80*	*Avg*		
1.	14.80	17.66	21.76	24.20	19.60	27.26	27.30	17.96	22.10	23.75	0	0
2.	15.93	18.80	20.06	21.63	19.10	16.43	23.60	27.30	25.06	23.50	1	0
3.	–	–	–	–	–	27.83	28.40	27.90	27.90	28.00	0	1
4.	–	–	–	–	–	6.00	23.00	14.53	23.56	18.02	1	0
5.	14.10	16.36	18.10	19.60	17.04	–	–	–	–	–	0	0
6.	19.13	21.06	18.90	19.73	19.70	9.10	9.73	9.43	9.20	9.36	0	1
7.	14.76	16.23	14.76	20.30	16.51	23.66	29.60	25.83	26.70	26.45	1	1
8.	–	–	–	–	–	19.16	7.03	7.33	29.76	15.82	1	1
9.	6.10	10.20	13.66	15.43	11.35	27.16	27.00	28.33	26.40	27.27	0	1
10.	–	–	–	–	–	26.40	29.96	29.53	27.96	28.36	0	1
11.	–	–	–	–	–	19.56	26.00	6.50	7.03	14.67	0	1
12.	–	–	–	–	–	6.00	6.13	8.96	9.46	7.64	0	0
Avg. act.	14.13	16.72	17.87	20.54	–	19.50	21.6	18.09	20.50	–	–	–

IP_1: Indicator parameter (=1) when alkyl group ($-CH_3$), $-C_2H_5$) is present otherwise (=0).

IP_2: Indicator parameter (=1) when two to three ring system is present otherwise (=0).

6 > 1 > 2 > 5 > 7 > 9 (4.5.1)

The reported Mannich bases (Table 4.5.1) are found more active against *K. pneumonae* in that only Mannich base **5** was inactive against the bacteria used. Here, the relative potential of Mannich bases against *K. pneumonae* is found as mentioned below:

10 > 3 > 9 > 7 > 1 > 2 > 4 > 8 > 11 > 6 > 12 (4.5.2)

However, the above eqs. (4.5.1) and (4.5.2) does not establish any QSAR between structure of the Mannich bases and their antibacterial activities against *E. coli* and *K. pneumonae*. Consequently, we have subjected the data to regression analysis using the method of least squares and obtained the most appropriate models using maximum R^2-method[28]. Because the number of Mannich bases active against *E. coli* and *K. pneumonae* are quite different, our discussion will be in two different parts dealing with *E. coli* and *K. pneumonae* separately. Below we first discuss the results obtained for *E. coli* followed by the discussion of results obtained in case of *K. pneumonae.*

4.5.2.1. Antibacterial Activity of Mannich Bases against *E. coli*

The topological indices (W, $^1\chi$, J, Sz) used for modeling antibacterial activities are shown in Table 4.5.2. In addition we have also used two indicator parameters IP_1 and IP_2 (Table 4.5.1). The indicator parameter IP_1 assumes the value of 1 when alkyl group is present in the molecule, otherwise IP_1 is taken as zero. Similarly, when two or more rings are present the indicator parameter $IP_2 = 1$; in absence of which $IP_2 = 0$. The intercorrelations of the topological indices, indicator parameters and their correlation with anti-bacterial activity against *E. coli* are shown in correlation matrix given in Table 4.5.3. The data show that W, $^1\chi$, and Sz are highly linearly correlated.

Table 4.5.2: Distance-based Topological Indices Calculated for the Set of Mannich Bases Used in the Present Study (Ref. Table 4.5.1)

Compound No.	*W*	$^1\chi$	*J*	*Sz*	*E. coli*	*K. pnenumoae*
1	10570	22.4257	1.5043	13258	19.60	23.75
2	9939	21.9257	1.5037	12186	19.10	23.10
3	9896	21.8591	1.5126	12259	–	28.00
4	11842	23.2134	1.5192	15486	–	18.02
5	9939	21.9257	1.5037	12188	17.04	–
6	7700	19.8532	1.9196	9368	19.70	9.36
7	3313	14.7322	2.6468	3832	16.51	26.45
8	3919	15.8082	2.1808	4480	–	15.82
9	6755	19.8772	1.3015	8402	11.35	27.27
10	4677	17.0248	2.6786	4677	–	28.36
11	4282	16.5213	1.8725	5752	–	14.67
12	11842	23.2134	1.5192	15486	–	7.64

W: Wiener index (Ref.17); $^1\chi$: First order molecular connecting index (Ref. 18); J: Balaban index (Ref.19); Sz: Szeged index (Ref.20,21), *E. coli*: Average activity; *K. penumonae*: Average activity.

Also that both W and Sz are highly linearly correlated with IP_2. Comparatively J and IP_1 with other molecular descriptors are less intercorrelated. Except IP_2, none of the remaining descriptors correlates statistically with antibacterial activity against *E. coli*. This means that no monoparametric model (except based on IP_2) could be obtained with statistical significance. That means we have to undergo multiparametric regression analysis for obtaining statistically significant model. Depending upon the data point (number of compounds used and active against *E. coli*) and in accordance with the "Rule of Thumb" we can at the most go for biparametric regression analysis.

Table 4.5.3: Correlation Matrix for Modeling Antibacterial Activity against *E. coli*

	W	$^1\chi$	*J*	*Sz*	IP_1	IP_2	*E. coli*
W	1.00000						
$^1\chi$	0.98058	1.00000					
J	–0.78196	–0.88380	1.00000				
Sz	0.99934	0.98323	–0.79342	1.00000			
IP_1	–0.39762	–0.48539	0.54268	–0.41295	1.00000		
IP_2	0.84281	–0.75330	0.50481	–0.83735	0.00000	1.00000	
E.coli	0.50190	0.33289	0.05932	0.49210	0.36172	–0.79041	1.00000

For details see footnote of Table 4.5.2.

Since the topological indices used are highly linearly correlated, the model based on combination(s) of any two of the topological indices may suffer defect due to collinearity. However, such cases are dealt very nicely by Randic[29] and we will use his recommendations while discussing such biparametric models containing highly linearly correlated topological indices. Consequent to this we have carried out biparametric regression analysis in two ways: (1) binary combinations of each of the topological indices with IP_1 and IP_2 respectively and (2) binary combinations of the topological indices themselves. The results obtained are present in Table 4.5.4.

A perusal of Table 4.5.4 shows that no statistically significant monoparametric model is possible for modeling antibacterial activity of Mannich bases against *E. coli*. However, the results do show that W and Sz are better for this purpose. The binary combinations of topological indices with IP_2 gave better results than those in which IP_1 is used as one of the correlating parameters. The topological indices W and Sz gave more or less similar results and that $^1\chi$ is better than both W and Sz for this purpose. The binary combination of J and IP_2 resulted into excellent models. That is, among the distance-based topological indices used J is found to be the best index. Earlier also we observed that J index is better than W, Sz and $^1\chi$ indices[32–34]. The best biparametric model containing J and IP_2 is found as below:

$$\text{Antibacterial activity against } E.\ coli = 12.8556 + 3.8064\ (\pm 1.2647)\ J - 6.1193\ (\pm 1.1369)\ IP_2 \quad (4.5.3)$$

$n = 6$, $Se = 1.2009$, $R = 0.9522$, $R^2_A = 0.8444$, $F = 14.567$, $Q = 0.7929$

Table 4.5.4: Regression Parameters and Quality of Correlation for Modeling Antibacterial Activity of the Mannich Bases against *E. coli*

TI (S)	*Se*	*r(R)*	R^2_A	*F*	*Q*
Monoparametric modeling					
W	2.9440	0.5019	–	1.347	0.1705
$^1\chi$	3.2100	0.3326	–	0.497	0.1036
J	3.3978	0.0593	–	0.014	0.0174
Sz	2.9631	0.4921	–	1.278	0.1661
Biparametric modeling based on combination of topological indices and indicator parameters					
W, IP_1	2.4033	0.7913	0.3768	2.512	0.3292
$^1\chi$, IP_1	2.8649	0.6846	0.1144	1.323	0.2389
J, IP_1	3.6077	0.3968	0.4043	0.280	0.1100
Sz, IP_1	2.4007	0.7918	0.3782	2.521	0.3298
W, IP_2	2.0876	0.8473	0.5298	3.817	0.4059
$^1\chi$, IP_2	1.8298	0.8857	0.6407	5.459	0.4854
J, IP_2	1.2009	0.9522	0.8444	14.567	0.7929
Sz, IP_2	2.0754	0.8492	0.5353	3.880	0.4092
Biparametric modeling based on binary combinations of topological indices					
W, $^1\chi$	2.0769	0.8616	0.57159	4.3355	0.4148
W, J	1.2695	0.9507	0.8399	14.1184	0.7489
W, Sz	3.1997	0.6244	0.0168	0.9586	0.1951
$^1\chi$, J	2.2825	0.8304	0.4826	3.3317	0.3638
$^1\chi$, Sz	2.2759	0.8314	0.4856	3.3595	0.3653
Sz, J	1.2815	0.9498	0.8369	13.8284	0.7412

For details see footnote of Table 4.5.2.

Here and thereafter n - is the number of compound, Se – standard error of estimation, R – multiple correlation coefficient, R^2_A – adjusted R^2, F – Fisher's ratio, and Q – quality factor. The quality factor Q is defined[30,31] as the ratio of R and Se (Q = R/Se) and account for the predictive power of the proposed model.

The coefficient of J in the above eqn. (4.5.3) is positive. This means that increase in the magnitude of J increases the antibacterial potential of the Mannich bases against *E. coli*. It is worthy to mention that the Balaban index J is a highly discriminating descriptor, whose value do not substantially increase with the molecular size and the number of rings present. Also, J is a variant of connectivity index; represents extended connectivity and is a good descriptor for the shape of molecules. As the coefficient of J is positive in eqn. (4.5.3) all these factors are favourable for modeling, monitoring, and estimating antibacterial activity of Mannich bases against *E. coli*. The coefficient of indicator parameter IP_2 is negative in the referred eqn. (4.5.3). We have used this indicator parameter IP_2 for accounting the presence of two or more rings in the Mannich base. Thus, the negative coefficient of IP_2 indicator that presence of two or more rings in the Mannich base is unfavourable for the exhibition of antibacterial activity against *E. coli*. As stated earlier because the effective number of Mannich bases used is 6, we can't go for still higher parameteric regression analysis.

We now discuss the biparametric regressions based on the combinations of topological indices alone. Such results are also presented in Table 4.5.4. At this stage it is interesting to record that with the development of several topological indices and their mutual correlatedness the questions arises: Is it proper to perform QSAR modeling using these highly correlated variables as descriptors. It is always necessary that selection of non-redundant descriptors is required. Fortunately such problem is nicely dealt with by Randic and that we will use his recommendations explaining the model containing such highly correlated topological indices and provide statistical justification.

The correlation matrix (Table 4.5.3) indicates that W, Sz, J and $^1\chi$ are highly linearly correlated. In addition, the W, Sz and $^1\chi$ are also linearly correlated. It means that all the models based on the binary combinations of these topological indices will suffer from the defect due to collinearity. Hence, we will have to use the recommendations of Randic for their justification and provide statistical evidence, if any, in support of such models containing highly correlated descriptors.

A perusal of Table 4.5.4 shows all the biparametric models containing some binary combination of topological indices, except for the model containing W and Sz, yielded statistically significant models. Out of these, the model containing W and J gave excellent results. The other model containing Sz and J is also found equally good. These models are found as under:

$$\text{Antibacterial activity against } E.\ coli = -11.6156 + 0.00172\ (\pm 3.0363 \times 10^{-4})\ W + 8.6607\ (\pm 1.8420)\ J \quad (4.5.4)$$

$n = 6$, $Se = 1.2695$, $R = 0.9507$, $R^2_A = 0.8399$, $F = 14.1184$, $Q = 0.7489$

$$\text{Antibacterial activity against } E.\ coli = -11.9358 + 0.00139\ (\pm 2.6835 \times 10^{-4})\ Sz + 8.9454\ (\pm 1.9039)\ J \quad (4.5.5)$$

$n = 6$, $Se = 1.2815$, $R = 0.9498$, $R^2_A = 0.8369$, $F = 13.8284$, $Q = 0.7412$

It is worth mentioning that Sz index is considered as the modification of W index for cyclic compounds. For acyclic molecules Sz index coincides with W index. Generally, Sz is found higher than W, while there are cases, in that Sz index equals W index. In the case of Mannich bases under present study in addition to cycles (aromatic moiety) the bases also contain acyclic (tree-like) side chains for which the coincidence of W with Sz is well known. Consequent to this, models containing W and J on one hand and Sz and J on the other hand have more are less similar statistics.

Before supporting our results using Randic[29] recommendations, we will like to discuss consequences of multicollinearity (other called autocollinarity). It is interesting to mention that the problems caused by multicollinearity, and how to deal with them, continue to be of prime concern to theoretical statistician. From a decision makers view point, one should be aware of that multicollinearity can (and usually does) exist and recognize the basic problems it can cause. Dealing with multicollinearity problems requires a great deal of experience. Some of the most obvious problems and indications of severe multicollinearity are:

(1) Incorrect sights of the coefficients,
(2) A change in the values of the previous coefficient, when a new variable is added for the model,
(3) Change to insignificant of a previously significant variable when a new variable is added to the model, and
(4) An increase in the standard error of the estimate when a variable is added to the model.

None of these problems exist in the models proposed by us (Table 4.5.4). It means that though theoretically the topological indices are highly correlated they perhaps contain hetero unknown information justifying their usefulness. This can be further elaborated using Randic recommen-dations. Randic[29] stated that selection of the descriptors to be used in QSPR/QSAR studies should not be delegated solely to the coacceptors although the statistical criteria will continue to e useful for preliminary screening of the descriptors taken from a large pool. Often in an automated selection of descriptors, a descriptor will be discarded because it is highly correlated with another descriptor already selected. But what is important is not descriptor parallel to one another, that is, duplicate much of the same structural information but whether they differ in those parts that are important for the property/activity considered both descriptors should be retained. If they differ in parts that are not relevant for the correlation of considered property/activity then one of them be discarded. Hence, following these recommendations of Randic the highly correlated topological indices are to be retained. We can do so again because none of the four problems due to multicollinearity, as mentioned above are present. In support of this finding one can use R^2_A values also. However, in the present case we could not do so as the highest multiparametric regression is the biparametric regression only. Use of R^2_A is more relevant, when we consider several multiparametric regressions starting from bivariant to the highest order of multiparametric regressions.

4.5.2.2. Modeling Antibacterial Activity of Mannich bases against *K. pneumonae*

We now discuss the modeling of antibacterial activity of the Mannich bases against *K. pneumonae*. Table 4.5.1 shows that in this case the sampling is rich as compared to the previous case of *E. coli*. Out of the 12 Mannich bases, 11 are found active against *K. pneumonae*. Based on the average value of the effective zone of inhibition following order of antibacterial power[35] is observed:

$$10 > 3 > 9 > 7 > 1 > 2 > 4 > 8 > 11 > 6 > 12 \quad (4.5.6)$$

However, this sequence doesn't establish structure-activity relationships. We have, therefore, subjected the data to regression analysis in that antibacterial activity was considered as dependent variable and the topological indices together with indicator parameters are taken as independent variables. The first step for such regression analysis is to obtain correlation matrix which provides information about mutual correlation between topological indices and their correlation with the activity (antibacterial activity in present case). In addition, we can use correlation matrix as a basis for undergoing multiple regression analysis. Such a matrix obtained in the present case of *K. pneumonae* is given in Table 4.5.5. This matrix is found more or less similar to the previous case of *E. coli*. Here also all the four topological indices are highly linearly correlated, thus arousing the defect due to colinearity. Also, that W, Sz and $^1\chi$ correlate highly with the indicator parameter IP_2 and that none of the descriptors used correlates statistically with antibacterial activity against *K. pneumonae*. Here also no mono-parametric models are possible for modeling the activity. We have thus to go for multiple regression analysis. Looking to the sample size and in accordance with the "Rule of Thumb" we can go upto triparametric regression analysis. As stated earlier we did so following maximum R^2 method and the results are discussed below.

Table 4.5.5: Correlation Matrix for Modeling Antibacterial Activity against *K. pneumonae*

	W	$^1\chi$	*J*	*Sz*	IP_1	IP_2	*K. pneumonae*
W	1.00000						
$^1\chi$	0.98892	1.00000					
J	–0.79296	–0.84938	1.00000				
Sz	0.99525	0.97987	–0.81269	1.00000			
IP_1	–0.10873	–0.19107	0.30922	–0.10131	1.00000		
IP_2	–0.80834	–0.76069	0.54225	–0.81243	–0.21429	1.00000	
K. pneumonae	–0.20547	–0.15823	0.08367	–0.25163	0.06586	0.22046	1.00000

For details see footnote of Table 4.5.2.

Although no mono-parametric statistically significant models are possible, we have reported the corresponding statistics in Table 4.5.6 as it gives an idea about the correlating powers of the descriptors used.

A perusal of Table 4.5.6 shows that in all the three cases statistically poor results are obtained. However, biparametric regression of topological indices yielded slightly better results, in that combination of W and Sz gave better results. Though, the statistics is not good it does give idea regarding relative correlation power of the topological indices used. In general this order is found as below:

$$Sz > W > {}^1\chi > J \qquad (4.5.7)$$

It means that the cyclic moiety of the Mannich bases play dominating role in the exhibition of anti-bacterial activity. The order: Sz > W also indicates that the tree-like (acyclic) side chain are less dominating in the exhibition of anti-bacterial activity of the Mannich bases used. Same is the case with $^1\chi$ and J, that is, first-order branching and extended connectivity are low, important in the exhibition of the activity.

In order to confirm our results we have estimated antibacterial action against *E. coli* and *K. pneumonae* using the best models. In case of *E. coli* we have used the models expressed by equations (4.5.3), (4.5.4) and (4.5.5), while the best model for *K. pneumonae*

Table 4.5.6: Regression Parameters and Quality of Correlation for Modeling Antibacterial Activity of the Mannich Bases against *K. pneumonae*

TI (S)	Se	r(R)	R^2_A	F	Q
Monoparametric modeling					
W	7.7712	–0.2046	–	0.3932	0.0263
$^1\chi$	7.8390	–0.1582	–	0.2310	0.0202
J	7.8994	0.0997	–	0.0903	0.0126
Sz	7.6836	–0.2516	–	0.6082	0.0327
Biparametric modeling based on combination of topological indices and indicator parameters					
W, IP_1	8.2345	0.2091	–0.1954	0.1828	0.0254
$^1\chi$, IP_1	8.2660	0.1907	–0.2045	0.1510	0.0231
J, IP_1	8.3159	0.1572	–0.2191	0.1013	0.0189
Sz, IP_1	8.1425	0.2549	–0.1688	0.2779	0.0313
W, IP_2	8.2048	0.2250	–0.1867	0.2132	0.0274
$^1\chi$, IP_2	8.2125	0.2209	–0.1889	0.2053	0.0269
J, IP_2	8.2074	0.2236	–0.1875	0.2106	0.0272
Sz, IP_2	8.1464	0.2531	–0.1699	0.2738	0.0311
Biparametric modeling based on binary combinations of topological indices					
W, $^1\chi$	7.8801	0.3525	–0.0947	0.5675	0.0447
W, J	8.2069	0.2238	–0.1873	0.2111	0.0272
W, Sz	7.1184	0.5342	0.1067	1.5973	0.0750
$^1\chi$, J	8.3026	0.1668	–0.2152	0.1145	0.0201
$^1\chi$, Sz	7.2483	0.5090	0.0738	1.3986	0.0702
Sz, J	1.2815	0.9498	0.8369	13.8284	0.7412

For details see footnote of Table 4.5.2.

was the biparametric regression expression containing W and Sz. The estimated values of the anti-bacterial activity are compared with their observed value. Such a comparison is given in Table 4.5.7.

In order to estimate predictive power of the proposed models we have calculated values for the quality factor Q (Tables 4.5.4 and 4.5.6). This quality factor Q is defined[30,31] as the ratio of correlation coefficient (R) to the standard error of estimation (Se). That is, Q = R/Se meaning thereby that the larger the value of R, the smaller the Se, the larger will be Q, and the better will be the predictive power of the models. Such Q-values corresponding to the models expressed by equation (4.5.3) – (4.5.5) are found as: 0.7929, 0.7489 and 0.7412 respectively indicating there by that the model containing J and IP_2 as the correlating parameters is not only statistically best but also has the best predictive power. In case of *K. pneumonae* the model based on W and Sz as correlating parameters has the highest value for Q, and thus the predictive power.

Table 4.5.7: Found and Estimated Antibacterial Activity of the Mannich Bases Using Regression Models for *E. coli*

Compound No.	Obs.	Models Based on					
		J, IP_2		W, J		Sz, J	
		Est.	Res.	Est.	Res.	Est.	Res.
1	19.60	18.58	1.02	19.59	0.01	19.95	–0.35
2	19.10	18.58	0.52	18.50	0.60	18.45	0.65
3	NA	–	–	–	–	–	–
4	NA	–	–	–	–	–	–
5	17.04	18.58	–1.54	18.50	–1.46	18.45	–1.41
6	19.70	14.04	5.66	18.25	1.45	18.25	1.45
7	16.51	16.81	–0.30	17.00	–0.49	17.07	–0.56
8	NA	–	–	–	–	–	–
9	11.35	11.69	–0.34	11.28	0.07	11.39	–0.04
10	NA	–	–	–	–	–	–
11	NA	–	–	–	–	–	–
12	NA	–	–	–	–	–	–

Obs.: Experimental value of the activity; Est: Estimated values using regression model; Res: Difference between observed and estimated activity; NA: Not active.

Table 4.5.8: Found and Estimated Antibacterial Activity of the Mannich Bases Using the Best Model Containing W and Sz Indices for *K. pneumonae*

Compound No.	Observed	Estimated	Residue
1	23.75	20.31	3.44
2	23.10	22.52	0.58
3	28.00	21.42	6.58
4	18.02	15.26	2.76
5	NA	–	–
6	9.36	21.91	–12.55
7	26.45	20.82	5.63
8	15.82	21.97	–6.15
9	27.27	19.72	7.55
10	28.36	28.69	0.33
11	14.67	15.06	–0.39
12	7.64	15.26	–7.62

It is worthy to mention that W and Sz indices are highly linearly correlated. Even then they can be retained in the models as they have different information contained. The W index is concerned with acyclic structure, while Sz is concerned with cyclic structure. Such a maintenance of W and Sz indices simultaneously in the model is in accordance with the recommendations made by Randic[29] and also in accordance with our earlier studies[32–34].

4.5.3. Conclusions

From the aforementioned results and discussion we conclude that the QSAR methodology used by us is better for *E. coli* as compared to *K. pneumonae*. Also, that a single topological index J, with IP_2 yielded better model and that the models based on the combinations of two topological indices are slightly worsed.

References

1. Tramontini, M.; Angiolinin, L., *Mannich Bases: Chemistry and Uses*, CRC Press, Boca Raton, FL, **1994**.
2. Tramontini, M.; Angiolini, L., *Tetrahedron Report Number*, 271, **1990**.
3. Joshi, S.; Khosla, N., *Bioorg. Med. Chem. Lett.*, **2003**, *13*, 3747.
4. Joshi, S.; Khosla, N.; Tiwari, P., *Bioorg. Med. Chem.*, **2004**, *12*, 571.
5. Joshi, S.; Khosla, N.; Khare, D.; Tiwari, P., *Acta Pharm.*, **2002**, *52*, 197.
6. (a) Khosla, N.; Joshi, S., *Acta Pharm.*, **1998**, *48*, 55.

(b) *Synthesis and Characterization of Some Mannich Bases*, Ph.D. Thesis (Navita Khosla), D.A. University, Indore, **1996**.

7. Joshi, S.; Maskar, S.; Khosla, N., Bhandari, V., *J. Indian Chem. Soc.*, **1997**, *74*, 156.
8. Joshi, S.; Khosla, N., *Indian Drugs*, **1995**, *32*, 398.
9. Joshi, S.; Khosla, N., *Indian Drugs*, **1994**, *35*, 548.
10. Khosla, N.; Joshi, S., *Indian J. Pharm. Sci.*, **1993**, 55, 198.
11. Dhaneshwar, S.R.; Khadikar, P.V.; Katiyer, J.C.; Dhawan, B.N.; Chaturvedi, S.C., *Indian J. Pharm. Sci.*, **1991**, *53*, 207.
12. Dhaneshwar, S.R.; Khadikar, P.V.; Katiyer, J.C.; Dhawan, B.N.; Chaturvedi, S.C., *Indian J. Pharm. Sci.*, **1990**, *52*, 261.
13. Dhaneshwar, S.R.; Khadikar, P.V.; Chaturvedi, S.C., *Indian Drugs*, **1990**, *28*, 21.
14. Dhaneshwar, S.R.; Khadikar, P.V.; Katiyer, J.C.; Dhawan, B.N.; Chaturvedi, S.C., *Indian Drugs*, **1990**, *28*, 24.
15. Dhaneshwar, S.R.; Khadikar, P.V.; Chaturvedi, S.C., *Indian Drugs*, **1990**, *27*, 431.
16. Dhaneshwar, S.R.; Khadikar, P.V.; Chaturvedi, S.C., *Indian Drugs*, **1990**, *27*, 625.
17. Wiener, H., *J. Am. Chem. Soc.*, **1947**, *69*, 17.
18. Randic, M., *J. Am. Chem. Soc.*, **1975**, *97*, 6609.
19. Balaban, A.T., *Chem. Phys. Lett.*, **1982**, *89*, 399.
20. Gutman, I., *Graph Theory Notes*, New York, **1994**, *27*, 9.

21. Khadikar, P.V.; Deshpande, N.V.; Kale, P.P.; Dobrynin, A.; Gutman, I; Dumotor, G., *J. Chem. Inf. Comput. Sci.*, **1995**, *35*, 547.

22. Kier, L.B.; Hall, L.H., *Molecular Connectivity in Chemistry and Drug Research*, Research Studies Press, Letchworth (UK), 1976.

23. Y.C. Martin, Quantitative Drug Design: A Critical Introduction, Marcel Dekker, New York (NY), 1978.

24. Kubinyi, H. (Ed.), *3D QSAR in Drug Design: Theory, Methods and Applications*, ESCOM, Leiden, The Netherlands, 1993.

25. Kubinyi, H., QSAR: Hansch Analysis and Related Approach in *"Methods and Principles in Medicinal Chemistry"*, Vol. VCH, Weinheim (GER).

26. Diudea, M.V. (Ed.), QSPR/QSAR Studies by Molecular Descriptors, Nova Science, 2000.

27. Karelson, M., Molecular Descriptors in QSAR/QSPR, *J. Wiley and Sons, New York, 2000.*

28. Chaterjee, S.; Hadi, A.S.; Price, B., *Regression Analysis by Examples*, 3rd ed., Wiley, New York, 2000.

29. Randic, M., *Croat. Chem. Acta*, **1993**, *66*, 289.

30. Pogliani, L., *J. Phys. Chem.*, **1996**, *100*, 18065.

31. Pogliani, L., *Amino Acids*, **1994**, *6*, 141.

32. Thakur, A.; Thakur, M.; Khadikar, P.V.; Supuran, C.T.; Sudole, P., *Bioorg. Med. Chem.*, **2004**, *12*, 789.

33. Khadikar, P.V.; Agrawal, V.K.; Karmarkar, S., *Oxid. Commun.*, **2004**, *27*, 17.

34. Khadikar, P.V.; Sharma, S.; Sharma, V.; Joshi, S.; Lukovits, I.; Kaveeshwar, M., *Bull. Soc. Chem. Belg.*, **1997**, *106*, 767.

35. Pharmacopoeia of India, 3rd ed. 1985, Govt. of India, Delhi.

Chapter 5
Summary

Mannich reaction provides an important biosynthetic route to natural products and several drugs. The most important application of Mannich bases is in the field of pharmaceutical chemistry. This is evident from the fact that more than 40 per cent researches concerning Mannich bases are published in Biochemical, Bioorganic, Pharmaceutical and Medicinal Chemistry journals. Literature has revealed that conversion of various acyclic conjugated styryl ketones into corresponding Mannich bases were often accompanied by increased bioactivity, both *in-vitro* and *in-vivo*. Various Mannich bases of chalcones and related compounds displayed significant cytotoxicity toward murine P388 and L1210 leukemia cells as well as towards a number of human tumor cell lines.

Consequent to above, our research group under the leadership of Dr. Sheela Joshi at Indore has synthesized a large series of Mannich bases of benzamides and screened them for their antimicrobial activity and toxicity. Similar type of work was also reported by another active group under the leadership of Prof. PV Khadikar. Both these groups of Joshi and Khadikar have also attempted qualitative structure-activity relationships supporting their results. However, no quantitative structure-activity relationships (QSARs) are attempted so for. This was, therefore, the primary objective of our Ph.D. work undertaken in the present study.

QSAR studies are based on a comparison between some type of activity and the chemical structure or physicochemical properties of a series of organic compounds acting as drugs. When a relationship between two chemicals is established, it can then be used to predict the activity of untested drug (organic chemical) of a similar nature. An extensive literature is available on such QSAR studies.

Two different schools mainly exist in the field of QSAR study. One school uses linear free-energy relationships very similar that of Hammett's and is the Hansch group. Prof. Hansch is considered as the father of QSAR. Consequently this group of Hansch uses parameters related to substituents, and thus doesn't give 1:1 correlation between structure and activity. The another group uses molecular descriptors called topological indices. These topological indices are numerical representation of the molecular structure. That is, in topological approach a structure can be represented by a number like activity. Unlike Hansch approach, this topological approach, therefore, gives 1:1 correlation between structure and activity.

An extensive work on the QSAR study based on topological indices has been carried by Khadikar and coworkers.

QSAR studies related to modeling antimicrobial activity of Mannich bases using topological indices appears to be an unexplored field. The objective of the present investigation, therefore, is to model more precisely antimicrobial activity of Mannich bases as prepared by Joshi and coworkers using distance-based topological indices. From the information thus generated, one or more lead compounds may be identified for subsequent development.

The study as reported in the present Ph.D. thesis is principally based on antibacterial screening and QSAR study of:

(1) Antibacterial activity of Nicotinoyl-4-aminobenzamidomethyl amines;
(2) Antibacterial activity of Mannich bases as compared to corresponding sulfonamides;
(3) Antibacterial activity of p-Nitrobenzoyl-4-aminobenzamido-methyl amines;
(4) Antibacterial activity of Mannich bases as compared to corresponding sulfonamides;
(5) Antibacterial activity of 3,5-Dinitrobenzoyl-4-amino benzamidomethyl amines; and
(6) Antibacterial activity of Mannich bases as compared to sulfonamides.

The antibacterial activity of the above systems will be modeled using some of the distance-based topological indices, such as following:

(1) Wiener Index(W);
(2) Molecular Connectivity indices (${}^{m}\chi_{R}$);
(3) Szeged Index(SZ);
(4) Balaban Index (J) etc.

Three bacteria *viz.* (i) *Escherichia coli*, (ii) *Klebsiella pneumonae*, (iii) *Bacillus subtilis* were chosen for the study. The data were subjected to regression analysis using the method of least squares. Finally appropriate models are proposed based on regression parameters and quality of regression.

The present Ph.D. thesis has been divided into four Chapters: I – IV, which deals with introduction and aim, topological concepts used in QSAR, topological indices used and results and discussion respectively.

In Chapter 1 a detailed information concerned with Mannich bases and their antibacterial activity is presented. Based on the survey of literature, the aim of the present investigation is given.

A detailed resume on the topological concepts as used in QSAR are presented in Chapter-II; while the details regarding topological indices are given in Chapter-III. This Chapter-III also presents the methodology used in developing QSAR models. In our study we have first used hydrogen-suppressed graphs in developing QSAR models. As in each of the Mannich bases there is a common molecular skeleton, we have then used rooted-graphs to develop QSAR models. The results herein are presented in Chapter-IV and a detailed comparison is made amongst the proposed QSAR models as obtained using hydrogen suppressed graphs as well as using those molecular graphs obtained from the rooted graphs.

The topological indices used in the aforementioned studies are: Wiener index (W), Szeged index (Sz), Balaban index (J), First-order molecular connectivity index ($^1\chi$), and logRB.

The results obtained are summarized in the following Tables 5.1 and 5.2.

Table 5.1: Results Obtained from the Hydrogen-Suppressed Graphs

No.	*Compounds*	*Best Model for Modeling Antibacterial Activity*		
		E. coli	*K. pneumonae*	*B. subtilis*
(1)	Sulfonamides	W, Sz	W	W, $^1\chi$
(2)	Mannich Bases: A Series (Chap.4.2)	$^1\chi$, J	$^1\chi$, J	J
(3)	Mannich Bases: B Series (Chap. 4.3)	Sz, J	W, $^1\chi$	W, Sz
(4)	Mannich Bases: C Series (Chap.4.4)	Sz, $^1\chi$	W, Sz	–

Table 5.2: Results Obtained from the Rooted Graphs

No.	*Compounds*	*Best Model for Modeling Antibacterial Activity*		
		E. coli	*K. pneumonae*	*B. subtilis*
(1)	Mannich Bases: A Series (Chap.4.2)	W, $^1\chi$	J, logRB	J
(2)	Mannich Bases: B Series (Chap.4.3)	W, $^1\chi$	W, Sz	Sz
(3)	Mannich Bases: C Series (Chap.4.4)	W, J	Sz, $^1\chi$	–

The results, therefore, show that the indices W and Sz play dominating role in modeling the antibacterial activities of the sulfonamides as well as the Mannich bases derived from them. The other important topological indices for such QSAR studies being $^1\chi$ and J. The details of the proposed models are given below.

Models Derived from Hydrogen Suppressed Graphs

(I) Sulfonamides

(1) Antibacterial activity against *E.coli*:

Antibacterial activity = 24.3154 + 0.0384 W – 0.0321 Sz

N = 5, Se = 1.1584, R = 0.9428, F = 8.001, Q = 0.8139

(2) Antibacterial activity against *K.pneumonae*:

Antibacterial activity = -1968.50+3.7250 W

N = 3, Se = 7.4458, R = 0.3781, F = 0.167, Q = 0.0508

(3) Antibacterial activity against *B.subtilis*:

Antibacterial activity = 94.2415 + 23.1249 $^1\chi$ – 0.1250 W

N = 5, Se = 3.3067, R = 0.8438, F = 2.472, Q = 0.2552

(II) Mannich Bases Belonging to A Series

(4) Antibacterial activity against *E.coli*:

Antibacterial activity = 23.6971 – 0.3575 $^1\chi$ – 4.5117 J

N = 12, Se = 0.8930, R = 0.4705, F = 1.2799, Q = 0.5269

(5) Antibacterial activity against *K.pneumonae*:

Antibacterial activity = -31.7149 + 1.4021 $^1\chi$ + 20.7946 J

N = 8, Se = 4.0435, R = 0.5864, F = 1.3101, Q = 0.1450

(6) Antibacterial activity against *B.subtilis*:

Antibacterial activity = 864.3680 – 790.6098 J

N = 3, Se = 0.7163, R = -0.9942, F = 85.103, Q = 1.3879

(III) Mannich Bases belonging to B Series

(7) Antibacterial activity against *E.coli*:

Antibacterial activity = 76.0813 – 0.0029 Sz – 30.5309 J

N = 6, Se = 4.8856, R = 0.6643, F = 1.185, Q = 0.1359

(8) Antibacterial activity against *K.pneumonae*:

Antibacterial activity = -19.0624 – 0.0039 W + 3.2120 $^1\chi$

N = 7, Se = 2.7867, R = 0.5372, F = 0.811, Q = 0.1928

(9) Antibacterial activity against *B.subtilis*:

Antibacterial activity = 7.3843 + 0.0100 Sz – 0.0131 W

N = 7, Se = 2.7882, R = 0.8116, F = 3.859, Q = 0.2911

(IV) Mannich Bases Belonging to C Series

(10) Antibacterial activity against *E.coli*:

Antibacterial activity = 63.1627 - 0.0038 Sz – 4.4148 $^1\chi$

N = 6, Se = 2.3471, R = 0.8196, F = 3.069, Q = 0.3492

(11) Antibacterial activity against *K.pneumonae*:

Antibacterial activity = 19.2228 + 0.0097 W – 0.00655 Sz

N = 11, Se = 6.7231, R = 0.6021, F = 2.2749, Q = 0.0895

Models Derived from Rooted Graphs

(V) Mannich Bases Belonging to A Series

(12) Antibacterial activity against *E.coli*:

Antibacterial activity = 11.9820 – 0.0013 W + 0.1734 $^1\chi$

N = 12, Se = 0.9568, R = 0.3261, F = 0.5353, Q = 0.3408

(13) Antibacterial activity against *K.pneumonae*:

Antibacterial activity = 1.2163 + 7.327 J + 0.0068 logRB

N = 8, Se = 4.2846, R = 0.5131, F = 0.8935, Q = 0.1197

(14) Antibacterial activity against B.subtilis:

Antibacterial activity = 351.8670 – 180.0464 J

N = 3, Se = 0.0913, R = -0.9998, F = 5288.94, Q = 10.94

(VI) Mannich Bases Belonging to B Series

(15) Antibacterial activity against *E.coli*:

Antibacterial activity = 4.3630 – 0.0549 W + 4.8174 $^1\chi$

N = 6, Se = 1.7506, R = 0.9635, F = 19.40, Q = 0.5503

(16) Antibacterial activity against *K.pneumonae*:

Antibacterial activity = 14.2453 – 0.0515 W + 0.0363 Sz

N = 7, Se = 2.7915, R = 0.5348, F = 0.8013, Q = 0.1916

(17) Antibacterial activity against *B.subtilis*:

Antibacterial activity = 9.6424 + 0.0074 Sz

N = 7, Se = 2.6546, R = 0.7831, F = 7.928, Q = 0.2950

(VII) Mannich Bases Belonging to C Series

(18) Antibacterial activity against *E.coli*:

Antibacterial activity = 2.9014 + 0.0043 W + 6.8633 J

N = 6, Se = 3.1272, R = 0.6459, F = 1.0738, Q = 0.2065

(19) Antibacterial activity against *K.pneumonae*:

Antibacterial activity = 18.2671 – 0.0054 Sz + 1.0047 $^1\chi$

N = 11, Se = 6.9572, R = 0.5634, F = 1.8597, Q = 0.0809

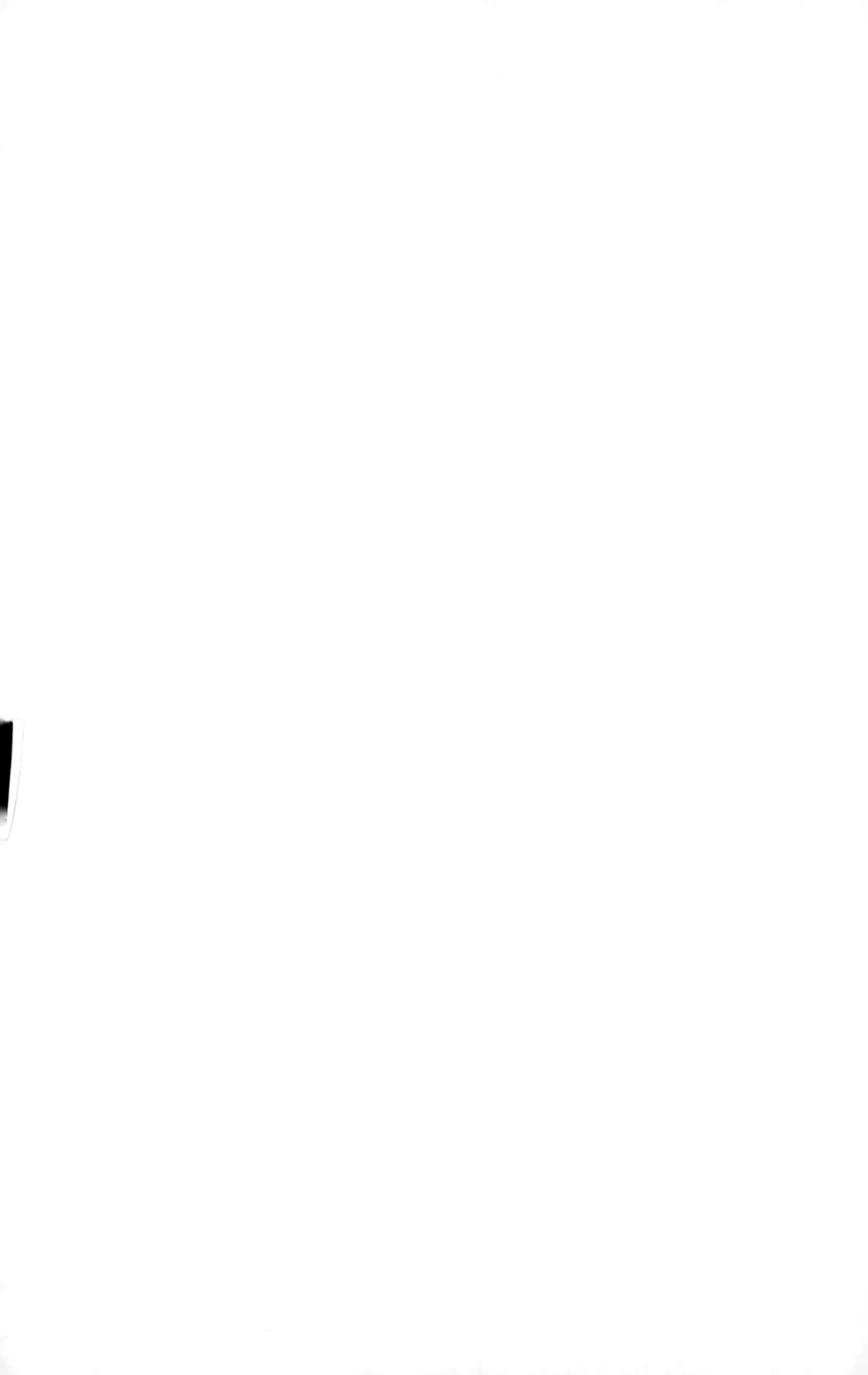

www.ingramcontent.com/pod-product-compliance
Ingram Content Group UK Ltd.
Pitfield, Milton Keynes, MK11 3LW, UK
UKHW021952270726
14060UKWH00002B/476

9 789351 309666